The Role of Eosinophils and Basophils in Health and Disease - An Integrated Overview

Edited by Jorge Morales-Montor

Published in London, United Kingdom

The Role of Eosinophils and Basophils in Health and Disease - An Integrated Overview
http://dx.doi.org/10.5772/intechopen.1008595
Edited by Jorge Morales-Montor

Contributors
Andrew Hudson, Aysu Timuroğlu, Claudia A. Garay-Canales, Cordelia Manickam, César A. Zavala-López, Diana L. Ruiz-Antonio, Hongmei Zhao, Jianmei He, Jorge Cime-Castillo, Jorge Morales-Montor, Karen E. Nava-Castro, Mariana Segovia-Mendoza, María del Sol Ríos-Avila, Neslihan Mandacı Şanlı, R. Keith Reeves, Raul Aragon-Franco, Valeria Vargas, Yair Rodríguez-Santiago

First published in London, United Kingdom, 2026 by IntechOpen
IntechOpen is the global imprint of INTECHOPEN LIMITED, registered in England and Wales, registration number: 11086078, 167-169 Great Portland Street, London, W1W 5PF, United Kingdom

For EU product safety concerns: IN TECH d.o.o., Prolaz Marije Krucifikse Kozulić 3, 51000 Rijeka, Croatia, info@intechopen.com or visit our website at intechopen.com.

British Library Cataloguing-in-Publication Data
A catalogue record for this book is available from the British Library

The Role of Eosinophils and Basophils in Health and Disease - An Integrated Overview
Edited by Jorge Morales-Montor
p. cm.
Print ISBN 978-1-83635-671-4
Online ISBN 978-1-83635-670-7
eBook (PDF) ISBN 978-1-83635-672-1

If disposing of this product, please recycle the paper responsibly.

Meet the editor

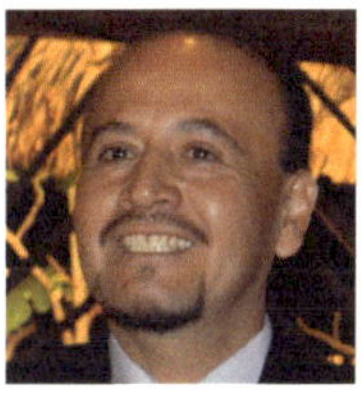

Dr. Jorge Morales-Montor's doctoral thesis was recognized with the Lola and Igo Flisser PUIS Award for the best graduate thesis at the national level in the field of parasitology. He received a Fogarty Foundation fellowship to conduct a postdoctoral research stay at the University of Georgia in the USA. He has 153 journal articles to his credit. He has also edited several books and written more than fifty-five book chapters. He is a member of the Mexican Academy of Sciences, the Latin American Academy of Sciences, and the National Academy of Medicine. Dr. Morales-Montor has won more than 35 awards and has graduated 35 bachelor's, 8 master's, and 12 doctoral students. He was previously the president and founder of the Mexican Society of Neuroimmunoendocrinology.

Contents

Preface

Eosinophils and basophils are two of the most common types of white blood cells, and have small granules that release enzymes when the immune system is under attack. This can happen during an infection, an allergic reaction, an asthma episode, or some chronic-degenerative diseases. Eosinophils and basophils form in the bone marrow and only live for a few days. Recently, it has become very clear that the roles of both eosinophils and basophils in many diseases are very important. Also, in normal conditions, they are key cells in controlling homeostasis. A lot of information has been published in the past few years around their role, for instance, in cancer, infection, and autoimmunity. This book focuses on chapters that examine the role of these cells in disease. Thus, this book aims to provide the reader with a comprehensive overview of the current state of the art in the role of a specific subset of immune cells, namely, eosinophils and basophils, featuring an easy-to-follow, vignette-based format that focuses on the most important evidence-based developments in this critically important field.

Thus, this book aims to provide basic and clinical evidence, based on molecular interactions and clinical studies, to address the roles of eosinophils and basophils in lung, viral, and cancer diseases, and to examine novel risk factors and the risks and benefits of novel immunotherapy.

Hongmei Zhao and Jianmei He, in their chapter *The Role of Eosinophils and Basophils in the Lung Health and Diseases*, discuss that eosinophils and basophils, traditionally recognized for their immune defense functions, have recently been shown to exhibit more complex roles in pulmonary immunity. Emerging evidence indicates that these immune cell populations not only protect the lungs but can also trigger excessive inflammatory responses when dysregulated. The precise roles of eosinophils and basophils in lung homeostasis and disease remain incompletely understood. This chapter comprehensively summarizes recent advances in understanding the contributions of eosinophils and basophils in acute lung injury, allergic respiratory diseases (asthma, hypersensitivity pneumonitis), and infection-related pneumonias (bacterial, viral, fungal). Authors critically analyzed both protective (immune surveillance and pathogen clearance) and pathogenic (exacerbating inflammation and tissue damage) dual functions with emphasis on cytokine secretion profiles, proinflammatory mediators, and granule release mechanisms. Special attention is given to their potential as a biomarker for clinical stratification. Translational evidence from murine models and human studies reveals critical knowledge gaps regarding tissue-specific activation thresholds and therapeutic modulation strategies. Furthermore, this chapter highlights promising therapeutic targets within eosinophil and basophil signaling pathways that could facilitate precision medicine approaches for respiratory disorders, ultimately proposing an integrated paradigm that reconciles their dualistic contributions to lung pathophysiology.

In the chapter entitled *Perspective Chapter: Eosinophils and Basophils in Lentivirus Disease*, Cordelia Manickam et al. discuss the role of these cells in lentiviral infections, which include human immunodeficiency virus (HIV) and simian immunodeficiency virus (SIV), that cause chronic immune activation, progressive immune dysfunction, and form persistent viral reservoirs despite effective antiretroviral therapy (ART). Authors note that while HIV research tends to focus on adaptive immunity or innate lymphocytes, the roles of granulocytic leukocytes, such as eosinophils and basophils, in lentiviral pathogenesis remain poorly defined. These granulocyte subsets, traditionally associated with allergic inflammation and helminth defense, possess a diverse repertoire of effector functions engaged in antiviral defense against HIV infection. These include direct cytotoxicity, antibody-mediated functions, the release of proinflammatory cytokines and chemokines, and the production of antiviral proteins, positioning them as important immune modulators in antiviral defense. However, their uncontrolled activation can also lead to inflammatory disorders and elevated risks for chronic diseases in people living with HIV (PLWH). Thus, the chapter reviews current knowledge and gaps in understanding of eosinophil and basophil biology in lentiviral infections, examines the cellular infection of HIV in these cell subsets, their activation and functions in HIV infection, and considers strategies to harness or modulate their functions in the design of vaccines and immunotherapies.

Valeria Vargas et al. delve into the roles of basophils and eosinophils in arbovirus infections. Authors state that arbovirus infections, including flaviviruses such as dengue and Zika, as well as alphaviruses such as chikungunya, continue to pose significant global health challenges. In the context of arboviral infections, innate immune cells, including mast cells, basophils, and eosinophils, play a pivotal role in their pathogenesis. This chapter aims to elucidate the roles of eosinophils, basophils, and mast cells as mediators between innate and adaptive immunity, highlighting their involvement in tissue damage mechanisms during infection and their contribution to stimulating both humoral and cellular immune responses. In certain instances, these cells may act as reservoirs, facilitating viral replication and dissemination within the host. A comprehensive understanding of these mechanisms has the potential to advance therapeutic, diagnostic, and prognostic strategies.

In the chapter *Perspective Chapter: Overview of Eosinophilia in Hematologic Cancers,* Neslihan Mandacı Şanlı et al. discuss that eosinophils are bone marrow-derived cells involved in the regulation of the adaptive and innate immune systems, tissue repair, and remodeling. If the absolute number of eosinophils in the blood is above $500/mm^3$, this is called eosinophilia. While eosinophilia frequently develops due to reactive (secondary) causes such as infection, allergy, and drug reaction, primary eosinophilia is caused by malignant clones in myeloid/lymphoid neoplasms. Life-threatening organ damage may develop due to eosinophil infiltration and granule release. The differential diagnosis of eosinophilia is quite complex and requires a multidisciplinary approach. Eosinophilia may also be observed in hematologic malignancies, and it is an important condition to consider in the differential diagnosis.

Finally, in the chapter *Eosinophils and Basophils in Breast Cancer, the Neglected Players?* Claudia A. Garay-Canales et al. present the role of eosinophils and basophils in breast cancer. Breast Cancer (BC) is the most common cancer and the leading cause of cancer-related mortality among women globally. This heterogeneous group of diseases can be clinically classified into three subtypes: luminal, HER-2, and triple-negative breast cancers (TNBCs). The immune system plays a pivotal role in the development and progression of cancer, with eosinophils and basophils being underestimated players. Although constituting less than 1–5% of circulating leukocytes, these cells can directly act on cancer cells via cell-surface receptors, releasing cytotoxic granule proteins and producing immunoregulatory mediators. Recent studies have shown that circulating eosinophilia and tumor tissue infiltration by eosinophils are associated with a favorable prognostic factor, particularly in patients undergoing concomitant therapy for HER-2-positive and TNBC. Immunotherapy, including neoadjuvant chemotherapy and immune checkpoint blockade, has demonstrated that elevated circulating eosinophils and tumor-associated tissue eosinophilia (TATE) are predictive of a more favorable treatment response. Although the study of basophils has been limited due to their rarity, emerging evidence suggests they play a role in various cancers, with ongoing investigations exploring their involvement in breast cancer. A more comprehensive understanding of the roles of eosinophils and basophils in breast cancer may facilitate the development of targeted therapies. The presence or absence of these cells in the tumor microenvironment could indicate the efficacy or failure of new breast cancer treatments. Further research is necessary to elucidate the mechanisms underlying the interplay between these immune cells and breast cancer.

We hope that our readers will find the first-ever book devoted to describing the roles of Eosinophils and Basophils in health and disease fascinating and enticing.

Dr. Jorge Morales-Montor
Full Time Professor,
Department of Immunology,
Institute of Biomedical Research,
National Autonomous University of Mexico,
Mexico

Section 1

Eosinophils and Basophils: Role on Disease

Chapter 1

The Role of Eosinophils and Basophils in the Lung Health and Diseases

Jianmei He and Hongmei Zhao

Abstract

Eosinophils and basophils, traditionally recognized for their immune defense functions, have recently been shown to exhibit more complex roles in pulmonary immunity. Emerging evidence indicates that these immune cell populations not only protect the lungs but can also trigger excessive inflammatory responses when dysregulated. The precise roles of eosinophils and basophils in lung homeostasis and disease remain incompletely understood. This chapter comprehensively summarized recent advances in understanding the contributions of eosinophils and basophils in acute lung injury, allergic respiratory diseases (asthma, hypersensitivity pneumonitis), and infection-related pneumonias (bacterial, viral, fungal). We critically analyzed their both protective (immune surveillance and pathogen clearance) and pathogenic (exacerbating inflammation and tissue damage) dual functions with emphasis on cytokine secretions profiles, proinflammation mediators, and granule release mechanisms. Special attention is given to their potential as biomarker for clinical stratification. Translational evidence from murine models and human studies reveals critical knowledge gaps regarding tissue-specific activation thresholds and therapeutic modulation strategies. Furthermore, this chapter highlights promising therapeutic targets within eosinophil and basophil signaling pathways that could facilitate precision medicine approaches for respiratory disorders, ultimately proposing an integrated paradigm that reconciles their dualistic contributions to lung pathophysiology.

Keywords: eosinophil, basophil, acute lung injury, allergic asthma, hypersensitivity pneumonitis, bacterial pneumonitis, viral pneumonia, fungal pneumonia

1. Introduction

As a core respiratory organ in direct communication with the external environment, the lung is continuously exposed to various harmful factors such as pathogens and allergens. These factors collectively contribute to the development of multiple pulmonary diseases, including acute lung injury (ALI), infection-related respiratory diseases, and allergy-related respiratory diseases [1]. Due to the high morbidity and mortality of these diseases, they have imposed a heavy burden on the global public health sector. Consequently, lung immunity research is pivotal for elucidating the pathogenesis of pulmonary diseases and advancing precision diagnosis and treatment [2]. Currently, there is an urgent need to deepen the understanding of the functions of eosinophils and basophils to support clinical translation. To resist pathogen invasion and maintain lung immune homeostasis, the lung relies on a complex network of immune cells to function—through the coordinated actions of various immune cells including pulmonary macrophages, mast cells, eosinophils, and basophils, the balance of the pulmonary immune microenvironment is collectively maintained [3]. Notably, as classical effector cells in type I hypersensitivity reactions, both eosinophils and basophils originate from common hematopoietic stem cells in the bone marrow. They can regulate immune responses by secreting inflammatory mediators such as major basic protein (MBP) and interleukin-4 (IL-4), thereby promoting the recruitment of immune cells [4].

Existing studies on eosinophils and basophils have gradually uncovered their key functional characteristics in pulmonary diseases. Taking eosinophils as an example, previous research on allergic diseases has clarified their life cycle: these cells undergo differentiation and maturation in the bone marrow before entering the systemic circulation [5]. In healthy individuals, the bone marrow produces an extremely small number of eosinophils, which not only results in a relatively low proportion of such cells in the circulation but also leads to a unique distribution pattern—they mainly reside in the intestinal mucosa and are presumed to maintain the homeostasis of the intestinal microbiota by participating in the regulation of the intestinal microecology [6]. However, when an allergic reaction occurs in the body, the number of eosinophils in the blood and tissues undergoes a significant change: Upon mobilization by inflammatory signals, these cells sequentially undergo adhesion, migration, and activation processes, ultimately infiltrating into inflammatory foci. At the foci, they release inflammatory mediators such as MBP and eosinophil peroxidase (EPO), which in turn cause tissue inflammatory damage, including alveolar injury, capillary leakage, and interstitial edema. This process is particularly critical in the pathological progression of allergic respiratory diseases and ALI [7]. Among these findings, the bidirectional interaction mechanism between eosinophils and type 2 innate lymphoid cells (ILC2s) holds considerable research value—type 2 cytokines secreted by ILC2s can induce the recruitment and activation of eosinophils, while eosinophils, in turn, enhance the activity of ILC2s, forming an inflammatory amplification effect that ultimately exacerbates asthma-related airway inflammation [8].

Similar to eosinophils, the immunological significance of basophils in the pathogenesis of allergic diseases has also been fully elucidated. These cells mature in the bone marrow and then enter the bloodstream to exert their effects. Circulating basophils can bind to IgE secreted by plasma cells *via* high-affinity FcεRI receptors, triggering a rapid degranulation cascade and releasing large amounts of inflammatory mediators, thus becoming a core driver of various allergic manifestations [9]. Recent studies have further revealed that during allergic reactions, a thymic stromal lymphopoietin (TSLP)/IL-4 signaling axis exists in basophils. This signaling axis not only activates Th2-type immune responses but also directly promotes the occurrence and development of airway inflammation, which is highly associated with the pathological mechanism of allergy-related respiratory diseases mentioned earlier [10].

Recent scientific advances have significantly expanded our understanding of the roles of these two types of granulocytes in pulmonary pathological processes, and they have shown important potential especially in the context of clinical translation. In the field of diagnosis, parameters related to eosinophils and basophils have become highly valuable biomarkers—for instance, absolute eosinopenia can serve as a prognostic indicator for the severity of coronavirus disease 2019 (COVID-19) pneumonia [11], while basophil depletion is associated with mortality in patients with community-acquired pneumonia (CAP) [12]. In the field of treatment, a number of innovative achievements have emerged: for example, GR30 (a licorice root derivative) can alleviate PM10-induced basophil inflammation by inhibiting the MAPK pathway [13], and remibrutinib, a Bruton's tyrosine kinase (BTK) inhibitor, is promising in suppressing basophil activation by downregulating CD63 expression [14]. These findings provide new directions for the precise intervention of pulmonary diseases.

Despite significant progress in research on the roles of these two cell types in pulmonary diseases, the field of translational medicine still faces many urgent challenges to address. At the diagnostic level, the insufficient specificity of single biomarkers makes it difficult to accurately distinguish between different subtypes of pulmonary diseases and to precisely assess disease severity and prognosis if relying solely on such biomarkers. At the therapeutic level, issues such as long-term safety monitoring of drugs and interindividual differences in drug responses still restrict the promotion of clinical applications. In this review, we will briefly clarify the dual mechanisms of action of eosinophils and basophils in ALI, allergic respiratory diseases, and infection-related respiratory diseases, and explore their translational value in diagnostic biomarkers and therapeutic interventions in combination with the latest clinical evidence, aiming to provide a basis for the precision diagnosis and treatment of pulmonary diseases.

2. Functional roles of eosinophils and basophils in pulmonary homeostasis

Traditionally, the accumulation of eosinophils in the airways has been considered a hallmark of allergic diseases and parasitic infections. However, recent studies have revealed that a small number of eosinophils are also present in healthy lungs [15]. Research by Loffredo et al. [16] demonstrated that eosinophils appear in the lungs as early as embryonic day 9 (E9), increase in number by postnatal days 7 and 14 (P7, P14), and subsequently decline to adult levels. This study also indicated that eosinophil numbers fluctuate during embryonic and postnatal development, correlating with specific stages of lung maturation. Further investigations by Mesnil et al. [17] identified two distinct eosinophil populations in developing lungs. Lung-resident eosinophils express transcripts associated with immune regulation and tissue homeostasis, capable of suppressing dendritic cell maturation *in vitro* and inhibiting allergic airway inflammation *in vivo*. Additionally, studies have shown that under physiological conditions, eosinophils predominantly localize to mucosal barriers including the gastrointestinal and respiratory tracts [18], where they perform essential roles in maintaining immune surveillance, facilitating tissue repair, and modulating immunomodulation [19].

As the least abundant granulocyte population [10], basophils have long been recognized for their contributions to immune regulation during allergic, infectious disease pathogenesis, yet their physiological functions in pulmonary healthy remained enigmatic until recently. Cutting-edge research by Schneidereit et al. [20, 21] have revolutionized our understanding by demonstrating that lung-resident basophils actively participate in the development and functional maintenance of alveolar macrophages through IL-33/GM-CSF-mediated signal pathways. This finding not only establishes basophils as tissue-resident immune cells but also highlights their critical regulatory role in lung development and homeostasis. Through sophisticated ligand–receptor interactions, pulmonary resident basophils engage in complex crosstalk with diverse cell types [22]. A particularly striking feature is their constitutive IL-6 production, implying functions extending beyond classical roles in TH17 differentiation and humoral immunity during lung development [23]. Moreover, lung basophils produce multiple cytokines and growth factors essential for the function of both immune and non-immune cells [22], profoundly redefining our conceptual framework of their multifunctional participation in respiratory system physiology.

3. Dual roles of eosinophils and basophils in pulmonary diseases

3.1 Functional roles of eosinophils and basophils in acute lung injury

ALI is a severe pulmonary disorder with high morbidity and mortality, the mortality rates up to 40% in severe cases. The pathophysiological hallmarks include alveolar-capillary membrane disruption, diffuse pulmonary interstitial edema, and gas exchange [24]. Emerging clinical evidence reveals a striking correlation between dynamic eosinophil counts and ALI patient survival rates, suggesting that evaluating the functional status of these cells may provide new insights for clinical diagnosis and treatment [25]. As an immunomodulator, eosinophils exhibit dual roles in ALI pathogenesis through cytokine networks and inflammatory mediator release. Beyond their classic pro-inflammatory mechanisms, recent studies have revealed their lung-protective effects mediated by immune defense mechanisms. Currently, research on the role of basophils in ALI remains limited, and their specific functions require further exploration.

3.1.1 Protective mechanisms: Eosinophils as immunomodulators

Contemporary research has uncovered a paradigm-shifting aspect of eosinophil biology in ALI, their capacity for tissue protection through sophisticated immunoregulatory mechanisms. Experimental models demonstrate that lipopolysaccharide (LPS) challenge induces a specialized CD101^{-} eosinophil subset that orchestrates pulmonary anti-inflammatory responses *via* promoting anti-inflammatory lipid mediators (e.g., protectin D1) production, thereby reducing lung injury and improving survival rates [26]. Additionally, IL-33 primed eosinophils exhibit enhanced protective capacity, effectively mitigating *Staphylococcus aureus*-induced ALI by reducing pro-inflammatory cytokine release, alleviating pulmonary edema, and decreasing neutrophil infiltration [27]. This finding collectively confirms a positive correlation between eosinophil accumulation and ALI survival, suggesting their role in modulating immune-inflammatory balance to counteract lung injury. In summary, eosinophils act as protective factors in ALI by exerting anti-inflammatory effects, mitigating pulmonary damage, and potentially improving disease prognosis.

3.1.2 Pathogenic mechanisms: The dark side of eosinophil activation

Under specific pathological contexts, eosinophils transition from protective sentinels to active contributors to pulmonary damage through multiple pathways. In the hemorrhagic shock induced injury, the HMGB1-RAGE signaling pathway triggers the accumulation of ILC2s in the lungs, leading to eosinophil infiltration and subsequent lung injury [28]. Besides, in LPS-induced ALI models, deficiency of activated leukocyte cell adhesion molecule (ALCAM) reduces inflammatory cell infiltration (including eosinophils), suppresses the release of cytokines (e.g., IL-1β, IL-6, TNF-α, CluOX2), and downregulates TLR4/NF-κB signaling, thereby attenuating lung injury [29], this finding suggest that eosinophils infiltration may promote lung injury. Similarly, in a superantigen-induced cytokine release syndrome model of extrapulmonary ALI, IFN-γ deficiency exacerbates ALI *via* enhanced eosinophil trafficking and IL-17A-mediated inflammation [30]. Furthermore, malathion inhalation has been shown to induce severe interstitial pneumonia, vascular injury, and marked eosinophil infiltration, accompanied by a significant reduction in pulmonary surfactant proteins [31]. These findings suggest that eosinophils may contribute to toxin-mediated ALI by releasing cytotoxic granule proteins (e.g., MBP, EPO) and amplifying inflammatory cascades. Furthermore, the observed functional diversity likely reflects microenvironment-dependent shifts in eosinophils subpopulations, the possibility that should be explored using single-cell RNA sequencing technologies in the future.

3.2 Functional roles of eosinophils and basophils in allergic diseases

Beyond the aforementioned dual roles of eosinophils in ALI, emerging evidence reveals functional heterogeneity of these cells across allergic diseases, including allergic asthma and hypersensitivity pneumonitis (HP) with distinct context-dependent behaviors, key research advances are summarized as following:

3.2.1 Allergic asthma

Allergic asthma is a common respiratory disorder characterized by airway hyperresponsiveness (AHR) and chronic airway inflammation. In its pathogenesis, eosinophils and basophils exhibit dual pro- and anti-inflammatory roles, often coexisting at allergic sites with potential crosstalk [32]. However, their precise mechanistic interactions remain unclear. Below we elaborate on their functions through immune defense and pathological inflammatory mechanisms.

3.2.1.1 The immunological defense roles of eosinophils and basophils in allergic asthma

In the immunoregulatory cascade of allergic asthma pathogenesis, inducible bronchus-associated lymphoid tissue (iBALT) orchestrates a multifaceted defense through three principal mechanisms: (1) potent suppression of eosinophil trafficking to pulmonary compartments, (2) delayed Th2 cell accumulation post-ovalbumin (OVA) challenge, and (3) dynamic reorganization of pulmonary T cell spatial architecture. This tripartite regulation culminates in diminished secretion of Th2-polarizing cytokines, particularly IL-5, the master regulator of eosinophil chemotaxis and activation, resulting in attenuated pulmonary inflammation and preserved tissue integrity [33]. Eosinophils paradoxically exhibit immunomodulatory sophistication in OVA/helminth co-infection models. Demonstrating unprecedented migratory precedence, these granulocytes infiltrate type 2 inflammatory niches ahead of lymphoid cells, independent of adaptive immunity. Mechanistic validation comes from IL-5/eotaxin$^{-/-}$ mice, where adoptive transfer of eosinophils fully restores Th2 competence for IL-13 production upon antigen rechallenge, establishing eosinophils as the bona fide regulators of adaptive Th2 immunity [34]. The immunological landscape reveals further complexity with the discovery of an IL-10^{+} ILC2 regulatory subset (ILC2s) in pulmonary mucosa. Defined by their cMaf/Blimp-1 transcriptional signature, these specialized cells establish autocrine-paracrine IL-10 feedback loops that quantitatively inhibit proinflammatory ILC2 effector programs. Functional studies demonstrate this subset's capacity to reduce AHR and diminish pulmonary eosinophilia [35].

Despite being the rarest granulocytes, basophils are potent regulators of allergic and anti-parasitic immunity. In the infection model induced by *Nippostrongylus brasiliensis*, pulmonary basophils secrete neuromedin B (NMB) to act on the NMB receptor on the surface of ILC2, inhibiting excessive type 2 immune responses through the "NMB-ILC2 signaling axis" and preventing destructive inflammation [36]. Furthermore, L. Bird's research indicates that in worm-induced lung injury, basophils exert a protective effect by inhibiting the cytokine secretion and proliferation of ILC2 [37].

3.2.1.2 The inflammation roles of eosinophils and basophils in allergic asthma

Eosinophils play a crucial pro-inflammatory role in the pathological inflammatory process of allergic asthma. The toxic granular proteins released by eosinophils, including MBP and EPO, can cause damage to epithelial tissues. Additionally, lipid mediators such as leukotrienes produced by eosinophils contribute to AHR and mucus hypersecretion. In the progression of allergic asthma, IL-33 can activate ILC2s, which produces type 2 cytokines to recruit eosinophils, thereby triggering airway inflammation [38]. Furthermore, the cytokine IL-13 released by eosinophils not only induces AHR but also promotes mucus hypersecretion by stimulating goblet cell differentiation. The released transforming growth factor-β (TGF-β) also plays a significant role in airway remodeling [39]. In house dust mite-induced allergic asthma models, different types of memory Th2 cells exhibit distinct pathological effects on eosinophils. Circulating memory Th2 cells migrate to the lung parenchyma upon stimulation, inducing perivascular inflammation and promoting eosinophil recruitment, while tissue-resident memory Th2 cells proliferate near the airways, activating airway eosinophils [40]. In allergic asthma, dysregulated type 2 immune responses lead to eosinophil degranulation, which induces tissue damage and airway hyperreactivity. Cytokines such as IL-5 and IL-13 are responsible for recruiting, activating, and regulating airway eosinophils. During type 2 inflammation, UDP-G activates P2Y14R on eosinophils, promoting their migration to the lungs, whereas inhibition of P2Y14R can reduce eosinophil infiltration and AHR [41].

In the presence of atopic dermatitis (AD)-like skin lesions, studies using a mouse atopic march (AM) model revealed that basophils play a critical role in OVA-induced pulmonary inflammation. In OVA-sensitized mice, basophil activation and IL-4 production were increased. Depletion of basophils alleviated eosinophilic pulmonary inflammation. Meanwhile, TSLP levels were elevated with topical MC903 application, and TSLP receptor knockout reduced pulmonary inflammation, indicating that thymic stromal TSLP is involved in basophil activation. Specifically, TSLP activates basophils to promote pulmonary eosinophilic inflammation in the AM model [42]. In allergic asthma, IgE readily binds to the cell membrane of basophils. When specific antigens interact with membrane-bound IgE, they trigger basophil degranulation, releasing immediate hypersensitivity mediators such as histamine, SRS-A, and PAF [43].

In summary, eosinophils and basophils are the key players in allergic diseases, and eosinophils release toxic proteins (MBP, EPO) and mediators (leukotrienes, IL-13) causing tissue damage, airway hyperreactivity, and remodeling, regulated by IL-5/IL-33/ILC2 axis. Basophils amplify inflammation *via* IgE/FcεRI-triggered histamine release and TSLP-induced IL-4 production. Their synergistic action drive type 2 immunity, making them prime therapeutic targets (e.g., anti-IL-5, P2Y14R inhibitors) for allergic disorders.

3.2.2 Hypersensitivity pneumonitis

HP is a group of interstitial lung diseases closely associated with environmental exposures, exhibiting significant heterogeneity in clinical manifestations, severity, and natural course [44]. Studies suggest that after specific inhalation challenge (SIC), patients with bird-related hypersensitivity pneumonitis (BHP) show elevated eosinophil counts and Th2 cytokines (e.g., IL-4, IL-5) in sputum [45], implying a potential role of eosinophils in HP pathogenesis, though the exact mechanisms remain unclear. Meanwhile, research on basophils in HP is limited, and their involvement is poorly understood.

Current evidence suggests that eosinophilic inflammation in HP may contribute to persistent inflammation and fibrosis in later disease stages. An increased eosinophil-to-lymphocyte ratio (ELR) correlates with poor prognosis, indicating a possible eosinophil/Th2-driven endotype in some HP patients [46]. Mitaka et al. [47] further support this notion, demonstrating that Th2-dominant responses in chronic HP sustain inflammation and promote fibrosis. Additionally, a study of three drug-induced pneumonitis cases revealed significantly elevated serum eosinophil counts and mild eosinophilic infiltration in lung pathology. Researchers hypothesize that eosinophilia may result from systemic hypersensitivity reactions or alveolar epithelial injury-induced cytokine release, facilitating eosinophil migration into the bloodstream [48]. Despite these findings, the precise role of eosinophils in HP remains unclear and warrants further investigation. Adam et al. [49] found that *Aspergillus fumigatus* allergens induce histamine release from basophils in HP patients. Since histamine promotes vasodilation and increased vascular permeability, basophils may exacerbate inflammatory responses in HP.

3.3 Functional roles of eosinophils and basophils in infection-related respiratory diseases

Eosinophils and basophils play complex and dual roles in infection-related pneumonia, participating in both anti-infection defense and pathological inflammation. The following sections summarize current understanding of the functions and mechanisms of eosinophils and basophils in viral- and bacterial-related pneumonia.

3.3.1 The functions of eosinophils and basophils in viral pneumonia

In viral pneumonia, eosinophils exhibit a dual role, including tissue inflammatory damage and antiviral affects. We discuss their functions in immune defense and pathological inflammation. Current research on basophils in viral pneumonia remains limited, and their specific roles in viral pneumonia require further investigation. Therefore, we mainly summarize the eosinophils' protective and harmful roles in viral pneumonia.

Eosinophils contain and produce antiviral molecules, including nitric oxide (NO) generated by inducible nitric oxide synthase (iNOS), which suppress viral replication through multiple pathways [50]. Eosinophils can recognize viral single-stranded RNA (ssRNA), double-stranded RNA (dsRNA), and DNA *via* TLR-3, TLR-7, and TLR-9 initiating immune responses to anti-virus [51]. Peripheral blood eosinopenia in patients correlates with poor prognosis, suggesting a protective role of eosinophils [52, 53]. Apart from the anti-virus function, eosinophils can also play pathological inflammation. For example, in severe COVID-19, eosinophil-mediated inflammation is heightened compared to non-severe cases. SARS-CoV-2 infection may drive specific innate immune responses, including eosinophil-mediated inflammation, and trigger subsequent lung pathology by enhancing Th2-biased immunity-potential a key driver of critical illness [54]. In a murine model of RSV-induced eosinophilic bronchiolitis, CCL11 (eotaxin-1)-mediated eosinophil recruitment to the lungs exacerbates disease severity [55]. RSV can induce eosinophils to form extracellular eosinophil traps (EETs) *in vitro*, potentially promoting airway obstruction [56]. Moreover, RSV-infected eosinophils can release infectious viral particles and pro-inflammatory IL-6 and aggravated the pneumonia progress [57].

3.3.2 The functions of eosinophils and basophils in bacterial pneumonia

In bacterial pneumonia, eosinophils and basophils also play distinct roles, yet their precise mechanisms remain incompletely understood. Eosinophils exhibit varying mechanisms depending on the bacterial species involved, primarily contributing to immune defense rather than pathological inflammation, though the exact regulatory pathways remain unclear. Studies using murine bacterial pneumonia models have demonstrated the antibacterial properties of eosinophils. Their cytoplasmic granules contain MBP and eosinophil cationic protein (ECP), both of which exhibit bactericidal effects. Additionally, toll-like receptors (TLRs) on the surface of eosinophils can enhance bacterial clearance [58]. In *Escherichia coli* and *Citrobacter rodentium* infection, eosinophils directly kill bacteria by releasing cytotoxic substances such as α-defensins [59] and reactive oxygen species (ROS) [60]. Eosinophils can also form extracellular traps that immobilize and eliminate bacteria, reducing bacterial load and protecting the host. Compared to eosinophils, research on basophils in bacterial pneumonia is limited, and their specific mechanisms remain poorly defined. Beyond bacterial pneumonia, increasing attention has been given to the roles of eosinophils and basophils in fungal pneumonia, atypical pathogen pneumonia, and tuberculosis, aiming to provide new insights for clinical diagnosis and treatment.

The dual mechanisms of eosinophils and basophils in various pulmonary diseases, including allergic asthma, hypersensitivity pneumonitis, bacterial pneumonia, viral pneumonia, and ALI—particularly the involved signaling pathways, inflammatory mediators, and cytokines—are systematically summarized as follows (**Figure 1**).

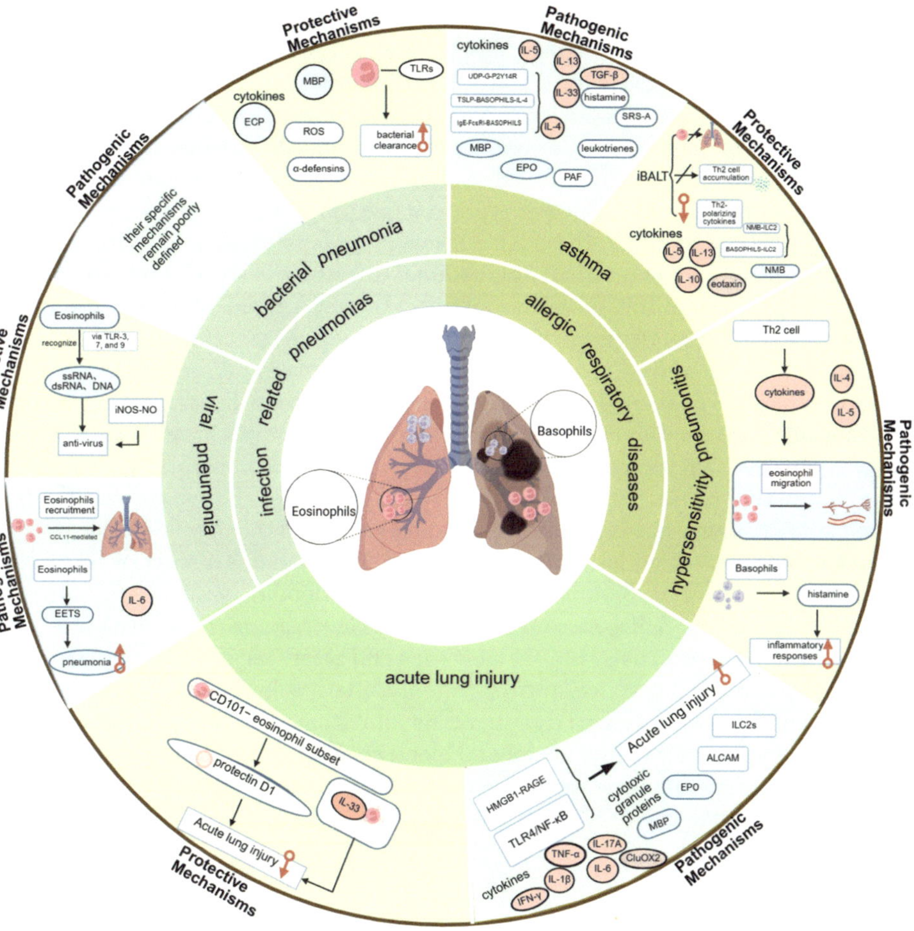

Figure 1.
Dual roles of eosinophils and basophils in pulmonary diseases. This figure comprehensively presents the protective and pro-inflammatory mechanisms of eosinophils and basophils across different pulmonary diseases, such as allergic asthma, hypersensitivity pneumonitis, bacterial pneumonia, and viral pneumonia—including pathways (e.g., TLR-mediated antibacterial pathway, IgE-FcεRI degranulation pathway), inflammatory mediators (e.g., MBP, histamine), and cytokines (e.g., IL-5, IL-4) involved. Created in https://BioRender.com.

4. Diagnostic, prognostic, and clinical translation potential of eosinophils- and basophil-associated biomarkers in pulmonary diseases

The previous sections reviewed the roles of eosinophils and basophils in ALI, allergic asthma, and HP. A common finding is that multiple inflammatory mediators and cytokines contribute to disease progression across different respiratory conditions. This raises the question: Do these factors possess diagnostic, prognostic, and clinical translational value? Below, we summarize existing biomarkers and their clinical applications, followed by a critical evaluation of emerging evidence.

For patients with ALI, emerging evidence suggests that peripheral eosinophil levels could serve as a valuable biomarker [26]. Monitoring this parameter can assist clinicians in evaluating disease progression and prognosis. In the clinical diagnosis and assessment of allergic asthma, the established biomarkers include allergen specific IgE (sIgE), total serum IgE (TIgE), sputum eosinophils, peripheral blood eosinophils, and fractional exhaled nitric oxide (FeNO), which collectively reflect disease characteristics and activity levels from different perspectives. Additionally, recent investigations have identified peripheral Th2 cells as a potential biomarker for predicting asthma exacerbations [61]. Furthermore, ceramides profiles have been confirmed as potential biomarkers for the diagnosis, prognosis monitoring, and therapeutic improvement of allergic asthma [62]. For HP, clinical studies have revealed that eosinophil count, monocyte count, and the ELR may serve as reliable prognostic biomarkers [46]. The comprehensive application of these biomarkers provides strong support for the precision diagnosis and treatment of allergic asthma. Currently, research on biomarkers for infection-related respiratory diseases remains relatively limited. However, preliminary findings have indicated an association between eosinophils and the severity of viral pneumonia [56], providing a foundation for future biomarker discovery in this field.

Beyond biomarker-related research, current studies on key inflammatory factors associated with eosinophils and basophils in respiratory diseases have also made some progress. However, interventions targeting these critical inflammatory factors remain in the clinical trial phase. For instance, in the pathogenesis of allergic asthma, the IL-33/ST2 signaling pathway has been confirmed to play a pivotal role, with IL-33 expression levels closely correlated with asthma severity [38]. Based on this discovery, researchers have developed several IL-33-targeting monoclonal antibodies, such as AstraZeneca's Tozorakimab and Sanofi/Regeneron's Ltepekimab. Nevertheless, these drugs are currently still in clinical trials, and their efficacy and safety require further validation. Additionally, in clinical practice, anti-IL-5 monoclonal antibodies (e.g., mepolizumab) have been widely used in asthma treatment. By inhibiting the biological activity of IL-5, these drugs significantly reduce peripheral blood eosinophil levels, thereby effectively controlling asthma symptoms and improving patients' quality of life [63].

5. Conclusions

Eosinophils and basophils play crucial roles in both pulmonary health and disease states. Under physiological conditions, eosinophils participate in lung development, tissue homeostasis maintenance, and immune regulation. In pulmonary diseases states, eosinophils and basophils assume dual roles of immune defense and pathological inflammation, manifesting in ALI, allergic respiratory diseases, and infection-related respiratory disorders. Significant progress has been made in mechanistic and clinical translational research, including the identification of biomarkers associated with these two cell types and the development of targeted therapies. However, numerous challenges remain, such as insufficient biomarker specificity, individual variability in targeted treatments, and long-term safety concerns. To achieve precision medicine, future research should further investigate cellular mechanisms, optimize biomarkers, develop personalized targeted treatment strategies, and strengthen clinical translation studies. These efforts will provide more effective approaches for the diagnosis, treatment, and prognostic evaluation of pulmonary diseases.

Acknowledgements

The authors are grateful to all the individuals who participated in this review. This study was supported by General program of Sichuan Natural Science Foundation (2024NSFSC0715).

Conflict of interest

The authors declare no conflict of interest and no financial disclosures.

Thanks

The authors sincerely appreciated the network support provided by the Gene and Cell Therapy Center, Institute of Blood Transfusion, Chinese Academy of Medical Sciences.

Appendices and nomenclature

MBP	major basic protein
EPO	eosinophil peroxidase
ILC2s	type 2 innate lymphoid cells
CAP	community-acquired pneumonia
BTK	Bruton's tyrosine kinase
ALI	acute lung injury
LPS	lipopolysaccharide
ALCAM	activated leukocyte cell adhesion molecule
HP	hypersensitivity pneumonitis
AHR	airway hyperresponsiveness
iBALT	inducible bronchus-associated lymphoid tissue
OVA	ovalbumin
NMB	neuromedin B
TGF-β	transforming growth factor-β
AD	atopic dermatitis
AM	atopic march
TSLP	thymic stromal lymphopoietin
SIC	specific inhalation challenge
BHP	bird-related hypersensitivity pneumonitis
ELR	eosinophil-to-lymphocyte ratio
NO	nitric oxide
iNOS	inducible nitric oxide synthase
ssRNA	single-stranded RNA
dsRNA	double-stranded RNA
EETs	extracellular eosinophil traps
ECP	eosinophil cationic protein
TLRs	toll-like receptors
ROS	reactive oxygen species
sIgE	specific IgE
TIgE	total serum IgE
FeNO	fractional exhaled nitric oxide

Author details

Jianmei He[1,2] and Hongmei Zhao[1,3*]

1 Gene and Cell Therapy Center, Institute of Blood Transfusion, Chinese Academy of Medical Sciences, Peking Union Medical College, Chengdu, China

2 Chengdu Medical College, Chengdu, China

3 State Key Laboratory of Complex, Severe, and Rare Diseases, Institute of Basic Medical Sciences Chinese Academy of Medical Sciences, School of Basic Medicine Peking Union Medical College, Beijing, China

*Address all correspondence to: hongmeizhao@ibms.pumc.edu.cn

References

[1] Kumar V. Pulmonary innate immune response determines the outcome of inflammation during pneumonia and sepsis-associated acute lung injury. Frontiers in Immunology. 2020;**11**:1722. DOI: 10.3389/fimmu.2020.01722

[2] Yong J, Shu H, Zhang X, et al. Natural products-based inhaled formulations for treating pulmonary diseases. International Journal of Nanomedicine. 2024;**19**:1723-1748. DOI: 10.2147/ijn.S451206

[3] Ryanto GRT, Suraya R, Nagano T. The importance of lung innate immunity during health and disease. Pathogens. 2025;**14**(1):91. DOI: 10.3390/pathogens14010091

[4] Kitamura Y, Yokoyama M, Matsuda H, et al. Spleen colony-forming cell as common precursor for tissue mast cells and granulocytes. Nature. 1981;**291**(5811):159-160. DOI: 10.1038/291159a0

[5] Lee JJ, Jacobsen EA, Ochkur SI, et al. Human versus mouse eosinophils: "That which we call an eosinophil, by any other name would stain as red". The Journal of Allergy and Clinical Immunology. 2012;**130**(3):572-584. DOI: 10.1016/j.jaci.2012.07.025

[6] Sturm EM, Knuplez E, Marsche G. Role of short chain fatty acids and apolipoproteins in the regulation of eosinophilia-associated diseases. International Journal of Molecular Sciences. 2021;**22**(9):4377. DOI: 10.3390/ijms22094377

[7] Davoine F, Lacy P. Eosinophil cytokines, chemokines, and growth factors: Emerging roles in immunity. Frontiers in Immunology. 2014;**5**:570. DOI: 10.3389/fimmu.2014.00570

[8] LeSuer WE, Kienzl M, Ochkur SI, et al. Eosinophils promote effector functions of lung group 2 innate lymphoid cells in allergic airway inflammation in mice. The Journal of Allergy and Clinical Immunology. 2023;**152**(2):469-485.e410. DOI: 10.1016/j.jaci.2023.03.023

[9] Karasuyama H, Miyake K, Yoshikawa S, et al. Multifaceted roles of basophils in health and disease. The Journal of Allergy and Clinical Immunology. 2018;**142**(2):370-380. DOI: 10.1016/j.jaci.2017.10.042

[10] Chen Y, Tang H, Yao B, et al. Basophil differentiation, heterogeneity, and functional implications. Trends in Immunology. 2024;**45**(7):523-534. DOI: 10.1016/j.it.2024.05.009

[11] Cazzaniga M, Fumagalli LAM, D'Angelo L, et al. Eosinopenia is a reliable marker of severe disease and unfavourable outcome in patients with COVID-19 pneumonia. International Journal of Clinical Practice. 2021;**75**(7):e14047. DOI: 10.1111/ijcp.14047

[12] Avci S, Perincek G. The alveolar-arterial gradient, pneumonia severity scores and inflammatory markers to predict 30-day mortality in pneumonia. The American Journal of Emergency Medicine. 2020;**38**(9):1796-1801. DOI: 10.1016/j.ajem.2020.05.048

[13]] Lee J, Ree J, Kim HJ, et al. Antiapoptotic and anti-inflammatory effects of an ethanolic extract of Lycium chinense root against particulate matter 10-induced cell death and inflammation in RBL-2H3 basophil cells and BALB/c mice. Plants (Basel). 2022;**11**(19):2485. DOI: 10.3390/plants11192485

[14] Kaul M, End P, Cabanski M, et al. Remibrutinib (LOU064): A selective potent oral BTK inhibitor with promising clinical safety and pharmacodynamics in a randomized phase I trial. Clinical and Translational Science. 2021;**14**(5):1756-1768. DOI: 10.1111/cts.13005

[15] Arnold IC, Munitz A. Spatial adaptation of eosinophils and their emerging roles in homeostasis, infection and disease. Nature Reviews. Immunology. 2024;**24**(12):858-877. DOI: 10.1038/s41577-024-01048-y

[16] Loffredo LF, Coden ME, Jeong BM, et al. Eosinophil accumulation in postnatal lung is specific to the primary septation phase of development. Scientific Reports. 2020;**10**(1):4425. DOI: 10.1038/s41598-020-61420-5

[17] Mesnil C, Raulier S, Paulissen G, et al. Lung-resident eosinophils represent a distinct regulatory eosinophil subset. The Journal of Clinical Investigation. 2016;**126**(9):3279-3295. DOI: 10.1172/jci85664

[18] Rosenberg HF, Dyer KD, Foster PS. Eosinophils: Changing perspectives in health and disease. Nature Reviews. Immunology. 2013;**13**(1):9-22. DOI: 10.1038/nri3341

[19] Lee JJ, Jacobsen EA, McGarry MP, et al. Eosinophils in health and disease: The LIAR hypothesis. Clinical and Experimental Allergy. 2010;**40**(4):563-575. DOI: 10.1111/j.1365-2222.2010.03484.x

[20] Schneider E, Petit-Bertron AF, Bricard R, et al. IL-33 activates unprimed murine basophils directly in vitro and induces their in vivo expansion indirectly by promoting hematopoietic growth factor production. Journal of Immunology. 2009;**183**(6):3591-3597. DOI: 10.4049/jimmunol.0900328

[21] Chhiba KD, Hsu CL, Berdnikovs S, et al. Transcriptional heterogeneity of mast cells and basophils upon activation. Journal of Immunology. 2017;**198**(12):4868-4878. DOI: 10.4049/jimmunol.1601825

[22] Cohen M, Giladi A, Gorki AD, et al. Lung single-cell signaling interaction map reveals basophil role in macrophage imprinting. Cell. 2018;**175**(4):1031-1044. e1018. DOI: 10.1016/j.cell.2018.09.009

[23] Yuk CM, Park HJ, Kwon BI, et al. Basophil-derived IL-6 regulates T(H)17 cell differentiation and CD4 T cell immunity. Scientific Reports. 2017;7:41744. DOI: 10.1038/srep41744

[24] Abdallah HM, El-Agamy DS, Ibrahim SRM, et al. Euphorbia cuneata represses LPS-induced acute lung injury in mice via its antioxidative and anti-inflammatory activities. Plants (Basel). 2020;**9**(11):1620. DOI: 10.3390/plants9111620

[25] Willetts L, Parker K, Wesselius LJ, et al. Immunodetection of occult eosinophils in lung tissue biopsies may help predict survival in acute lung injury. Respiratory Research. 2011;**12**(1):116. DOI: 10.1186/1465-9921-12-116

[26] Zhu C, Weng QY, Zhou LR, et al. Homeostatic and earlyrecruited CD101(−) eosinophils suppress endotoxin-induced acute lung injury. The European Respiratory Journal. 2020;**56**(5):1902354. DOI: 10.1183/13993003.02354-2019

[27] Krishack PA, Hollinger MK, Kuzel TG, et al. IL-33-mediated eosinophilia protects against acute lung injury. American Journal of Respiratory Cell and Molecular Biology. 2021;**64**(5):569-578. DOI: 10.1165/rcmb.2020-0166OC

[28] Zhang K, Jin Y, Lai D, et al. RAGE-induced ILC2 expansion in

acute lung injury due to haemorrhagic shock. Thorax. 2020;**75**(3):209-219. DOI: 10.1136/thoraxjnl-2019-213613

[29] Li R, Ren T, Zeng J, et al. ALCAM deficiency alleviates LPS-induced acute lung injury by inhibiting inflammatory response. Inflammation. 2023;**46**(2):688-699. DOI: 10.1007/s10753-022-01765-3

[30] Sun Y, Hu B, Stanley G, et al. IFN-γ is protective in cytokine release syndrome-associated extrapulmonary acute lung injury. American Journal of Respiratory Cell and Molecular Biology. 2023;**68**(1):75-89. DOI: 10.1165/rcmb.2022-0117OC

[31] Abdo W, Elmadawy MA, Abdelhiee EY, et al. Protective effect of thymoquinone against lung intoxication induced by malathion inhalation. Scientific Reports. 2021;**11**(1):2498. DOI: 10.1038/s41598-021-82083-w

[32] Iype J, Fux M. Basophils orchestrating eosinophils' chemotaxis and function in allergic inflammation. Cells. 2021;**10**(4):895. DOI: 10.3390/cells10040895

[33] Hwang JY, Silva-Sanchez A, Carragher DM, et al. Inducible bronchus-associated lymphoid tissue (iBALT) attenuates pulmonary pathology in a mouse model of allergic airway disease. Frontiers in Immunology. 2020;**11**:570661. DOI: 10.3389/fimmu.2020.570661

[34] Kita H. Eosinophils: Multifaceted biological properties and roles in health and disease. Immunological Reviews. 2011;**242**(1):161-177. DOI: 10.1111/j.1600-065X.2011.01026.x

[35] Howard E, Lewis G, Galle-Treger L, et al. IL-10 production by ILC2s requires Blimp-1 and cMaf, modulates cellular metabolism, and ameliorates airway hyperreactivity. The Journal of Allergy and Clinical Immunology. 2021;**147**(4):1281-1295.e1285. DOI: 10.1016/j.jaci.2020.08.024

[36] Inclan-Rico JM, Ponessa JJ, Valero-Pacheco N, et al. Basophils prime group 2 innate lymphoid cells for neuropeptide-mediated inhibition. Nature Immunology. 2020;**21**(10):1181-1193. DOI: 10.1038/s41590-020-0753-y

[37] Bird L. Basophils balance ILC2s. Nature Reviews. Immunology. 2020;**20**(10):592-593. DOI: 10.1038/s41577-020-00437-3

[38] Liew FY, Girard JP, Turnquist HR. Interleukin-33 in health and disease. Nature Reviews. Immunology. 2016;**16**(11):676-689. DOI: 10.1038/nri.2016.95

[39] McBrien CN, Menzies-Gow A. The biology of eosinophils and their role in asthma. Frontiers in Medicine (Lausanne). 2017;**4**:93. DOI: 10.3389/fmed.2017.00093

[40] Rahimi RA, Nepal K, Cetinbas M, et al. Distinct functions of tissue-resident and circulating memory Th2 cells in allergic airway disease. The Journal of Experimental Medicine. 2020;**217**(9):e20190865. DOI: 10.1084/jem.2019086

[41] Foster PS, Tay HL, Hogan SP. Uridine diphosphate-glucose/P2Y14R axis is a nonchemokine pathway that selectively promotes eosinophil accumulation. The Journal of Clinical Investigation. 2021;**131**(7):e147735. DOI: 10.1172/jci147735

[42] Li X, Li Z, Tang M, et al. Thymic stromal lymphopoietin-activated basophil promotes lung inflammation in mouse atopic march model. Frontiers in Immunology. 2025;**16**:1573130. DOI: 10.3389/fimmu.2025.1573130

[43] Sticco KL, Pandya NK, Zubair M, et al. *Basophilia*. In: StatPearls. Treasure Island (FL): StatPearls Publishing LLC; 2025

[44] Vasakova M, Selman M, Morell F, et al. Hypersensitivity pneumonitis: Current concepts of pathogenesis and potential targets for treatment. American Journal of Respiratory and Critical Care Medicine. 2019;**200**(3):301-308. DOI: 10.1164/rccm.201903-0541PP

[45] Villar A, Muñoz X, Sanchez-Vidaurre S, et al. Bronchial inflammation in hypersensitivity pneumonitis after antigen-specific inhalation challenge. Respirology. 2014;**19**(6):891-899. DOI: 10.1111/resp.12323

[46] Katsaras M, Sotiropoulou V, Manali E, et al. Complete blood cell count parameters predict mortality in patients with hypersensitivity pneumonitis. Diagnostics (Basel). 2025;**15**(8):1038. DOI: 10.3390/diagnostics15081038

[47] Mitaka K, Miyazaki Y, Yasui M, et al. Th2-biased immune responses are important in a murine model of chronic hypersensitivity pneumonitis. International Archives of Allergy and Immunology. 2011;**154**(3):264-274. DOI: 10.1159/000321114

[48] Kaneko T, Otoshi R, Sekine A, et al. Drug-related pneumonitis caused by amikacin liposome inhalation suspension: One pathologically proven case and single-center experience. Respiratory Investigation. 2024;**62**(4):513-516. DOI: 10.1016/j.resinv.2024.04.003

[49] Adam J, Graf LM, Westermann S, et al. Signaling events driving *Aspergillus fumigatus*-induced eosinophil activation. International Journal of Medical Microbiology. 2025;**318**:151641. DOI: 10.1016/j.ijmm.2024.151641

[50] Abdul-Cader MS, Amarasinghe A, Abdul-Careem MF. Activation of toll-like receptor signaling pathways leading to nitric oxide-mediated antiviral responses. Archives of Virology. 2016;**161**(8):2075-2086. DOI: 10.1007/s00705-016-2904-x

[51] Kvarnhammar AM, Cardell LO. Pattern-recognition receptors in human eosinophils. Immunology. 2012;**136**(1):11-20. DOI: 10.1111/j.1365-2567.2012.03556.x

[52] Tanni F, Akker E, Zaman MM, et al. Eosinopenia and COVID-19. The Journal of the American Osteopathic Association. 2020. DOI: 10.7556/jaoa.2020.091.Online ahead of print

[53] Morais-Almeida M, Aguiar R, Martin B, et al. COVID-19, asthma, and biological therapies: What we need to know. World Allergy Organization Journal. 2020;**13**(5):100126. DOI: 10.1016/j.waojou.2020.100126

[54] Kim DM, Kim Y, Seo JW, et al. Enhanced eosinophil-mediated inflammation associated with antibody and complement-dependent pneumonic insults in critical COVID-19. Cell Reports. 2021;**37**(1):109798. DOI: 10.1016/j.celrep.2021.109798

[55] Matthews SP, Tregoning JS, Coyle AJ, et al. Role of CCL11 in eosinophilic lung disease during respiratory syncytial virus infection. Journal of Virology. 2005;**79**(4):2050-2057. DOI: 10.1128/jvi.79.4.2050-2057.2005

[56] Silveira JS, Antunes GL, Gassen RB, et al. Respiratory syncytial virus increases eosinophil extracellular traps in a murine model of asthma. Asia Pacific Allergy. 2019;**9**(4):e32. DOI: 10.5415/apallergy.2019.9.e32

[57] Dyer KD, Percopo CM, Fischer ER, et al. Pneumoviruses

infect eosinophils and elicit MyD88-dependent release of chemoattractant cytokines and interleukin-6. Blood. 2009;**114**(13):2649-2656. DOI: 10.1182/blood-2009-01-199497

[58] Linch SN, Kelly AM, Danielson ET, et al. Mouse eosinophils possess potent antibacterial properties in vivo. Infection and Immunity. 2009;**77**(11):4976-4982. DOI: 10.1128/iai.00306-09

[59] Khatun A, Sakurai M, Sakai Y, et al. Mycobacterial infection induces eosinophilia and production of α-defensin by eosinophils in mice. The Journal of Veterinary Medical Science. 2019;**81**(1):138-142. DOI: 10.1292/jvms.18-0619

[60] Driss V, Legrand F, Hermann E, et al. TLR2-dependent eosinophil interactions with mycobacteria: Role of alpha-defensins. Blood. 2009;**113**(14):3235-3244. DOI: 10.1182/blood-2008-07-166595

[61] Shrestha Palikhe N, Wu Y, Konrad E, et al. Th2 cell markers in peripheral blood increase during an acute asthma exacerbation. Allergy. 2021;**76**(1):281-290. DOI: 10.1111/all.14543

[62] James BN, Oyeniran C, Sturgill JL, et al. Ceramide in apoptosis and oxidative stress in allergic inflammation and asthma. The Journal of Allergy and Clinical Immunology. 2021;**147**(5):1936-1948.e1939. DOI: 10.1016/j.jaci.2020.10.024

[63] Busse WW, Ring J, Huss-Marp J, et al. A review of treatment with mepolizumab, an anti-IL-5 mAb, in hypereosinophilic syndromes and asthma. The Journal of Allergy and Clinical Immunology. 2010;**125**(4):803-813. DOI: 10.1016/j.jaci.2009.11.048

Section 2

Eosinophils and Basophils in Virus Infections

Chapter 2

Perspective Chapter: Eosinophils and Basophils in Lentivirus Disease

Cordelia Manickam, Andrew Hudson and R. Keith Reeves

Abstract

Lentiviral infections which include human immunodeficiency virus (HIV) and simian immunodeficiency virus (SIV) cause chronic immune activation, progressive immune dysfunction and form persistent viral reservoirs despite effective antiretroviral therapy (ART). While HIV research tends to focus on adaptive immunity or innate lymphocytes, the roles granulocytic leukocytes, such as eosinophils and basophils, in lentiviral pathogenesis remain poorly defined. These granulocyte subsets, traditionally associated with allergic inflammation and helminth defense, possess a diverse repertoire of effector functions engaged in antiviral defense against HIV infection These include direct cytotoxicity, antibody-mediated functions, and the release of pro-inflammatory cytokines and chemokines, as well as antiviral proteins, positioning them as important immune modulators in antiviral defense. However, their uncontrolled activation can also lead to inflammatory disorders and elevated risks for chronic diseases in people living with HIV (PLWH). This chapter reviews current knowledge and gaps in understanding of eosinophil and basophil biology in lentiviral infections, examines the cellular infection of HIV in these cell subsets, their activation and functions in HIV infection and considers strategies to harness or modulate their functions in the design of vaccines and immunotherapies.

Keywords: eosinophil, basophil, lentivirus, HIV immunity, granulocyte, innate immunity

1. Introduction

Eosinophils and basophils are important innate effector cells that help defend the body from pathogens but also regulate allergic responses. They are granulocytic immune cells that arise from a shared myeloid progenitor and possess an arsenal of effector mechanisms including cytotoxic granule proteins, secretion of cytokines and chemokines, generation of reactive oxygen species and formation of extracellular traps. They also express a diverse repertoire of Fc receptors and pattern recognition receptors which makes them critical effectors of antibody- dependent functions. They modulate inflammatory milieus and can crosstalk with other innate and adaptive immune cells, thus shaping immune outcomes. But while they are well established as potent mediators and effectors in allergic and parasitic infections their antiviral activities, particularly in the context of lentiviral infections, remain underexplored.

Human Immunodeficiency virus (HIV) is the most clinically significant lentiviral infection, responsible for global pandemic recognized since the early 1980s. Despite major advances in prevention, diagnosis and treatment to suppress viral replication through antiretroviral therapy (ART), HIV remains a major global health challenge. Persistent viral reservoirs, chronic immune activation and a myriad of multiple comorbid conditions continue to affect and lower the quality of life in people living with HIV (PLWH). While extensive research has focused on adaptive immunity and innate effectors such as macrophages, NK cells, and neutrophils, comparatively little is known about the contributions of eosinophils and basophils in lentiviral pathologies. Understanding their roles could reveal novel pathways to modulate immune responses in the context of HIV infection, vaccination and therapeutic intervention. In this chapter, we review the current understanding of eosinophil and basophil biology in the context of HIV infection, highlighting both established findings and unresolved questions. We identify critical gaps in knowledge and discuss how we can harness these cells for enhancing anti-HIV immunity.

2. HIV- The virus and the disease

HIV is responsible for the continuing acquired immunodeficiency syndrome (AIDS) epidemic which began in the early 1980s [1, 2]. HIV emerged in the early twentieth century in Africa by zoonotic transmission from chimpanzees, and ultimately derives from Simian Immunodeficiency Virus (SIV), which is found in several African non-human primate species [3]. As of a 2023 WHO report, there were approximately 39.9 million people were living with HIV worldwide in 2023 [4]. HIV is transmitted by several bodily fluids, including blood, breast milk, and semen, and is a sexually transmitted disease [5]. There are two distantly related types of HIV, HIV-1 and HIV-2, with the latter localized to regions of southern Africa, exhibiting a lower degree of transmissibility and morbidity than HIV-1 [3]. Since the beginning of the epidemic, HIV/AIDS has represented a global health crisis and claimed over forty million lives. While historic progress has been made toward anti-retroviral therapy (ART) which prevents viral replication and improves the quality of life, PLWH are still at increased risk for various co-morbidities including cardiovascular disease, chronic kidney and liver diseases, and certain types of cancer [6, 7]. Currently, there is no broadly effective prophylactic HIV vaccine or curative therapy, and the cost and inconvenience of existing therapeutics create a barrier for uptake, especially in communities that are most affected [6, 8, 9].

HIV belongs to the genus *Lentivirus* in the family *Retroviridae*. The HIV virion is composed of a lipid envelope embedded with glycoproteins that surrounds a protein capsid, which in turn contains a nucleocapsid associated with viral RNA [2]. The HIV envelope proteins bind to CD4 and one of two coreceptors, CCR5 or CXCR4 depending on viral tropism, in order to fuse with the cell surface and enter the cell. Following virion fusion, viral RNA and proteins enter the cytoplasm, and reverse transcriptase converts the RNA genome into DNA [2]. These new DNA genomes integrate into host chromosomes via integrases, where they drive viral replication and capsid production, eventually releasing new virions into the environment [2]. The result is a steady depletion of CD4+ T cells that leads to weakened immune competence and vulnerability to secondary infections [2, 10]. The median survival time for individuals with untreated HIV is between 8 and 10 years [10].

In the late 1980s, Azidothymidine (AZT) was developed as the first of many antiretroviral drugs, which acted by inhibiting HIV replication. AZT alone was unable to suppress the virus long-term, but as more antiretrovirals were developed, combination antiretroviral therapies (cARTs) emerged as the dominant treatment strategy [6, 11]. Today, cART treatments can consistently suppress HIV viral loads to sub-symptomatic and non-transmittable levels [6]. However, cART is unable to cure HIV due to several factors. Firstly, infected cells frequently enter a state of latency, in which the viral DNA inserted into the genome, called a provirus, ceases expression of viral elements [11]. These latently infected cells persist despite ART, in circulation as well as in tissue reservoirs such as the spleen, lymph nodes, and gut [12]. HIV provirus sporadically re-activates, causing viral load to rebound in patients removed from ART treatment [11, 12]. Secondly, HIV rapidly mutates within the host, and selective pressure from ART constantly spurs ART-resistant adaptations that necessitate the cycling of different combination antiretrovirals [13]. For these reasons, the development of an HIV cure will require strategies beyond cART alone, such as cell-based therapeutics or "shock and kill" therapies - a term for the combination of latency-reversing drugs to "awaken" provirus alongside antivirals to eliminate infected cells [14]. While a cure may be years away, substantial progress has been made toward HIV prevention with the advent of Pre-Exposure Prophylaxis (PrEP) drugs for HIV, with the first having been approved by the FDA in 2012 [15]. Notably, socioeconomic factors continue to limit PrEP usage in at-risk communities [9].

Achieving a solution to HIV will require a comprehensive understanding and strategic modulation of the immune environment in the context of infection. HIV not only compromises immune function by lowering CD4+ T cell counts, but also promotes systemic inflammation, triggering overactivation and exhaustion across a wide variety of immune cell types [16, 17]. HIV increases CD8+ T cell frequency regardless of ART treatment, raising the risk for inflammatory pathologies. In some instances, elite controllers (ECs) naturally suppress viral levels due to robust HIV-specific CD8+ T cell response, suggesting a potential role for cytotoxic T cells in future therapeutics [16, 18]. CD4+ T cell subsets vary widely in their impact on HIV; existing Th1 populations shift toward a Th2 state throughout the course of infection, skewing the immune landscape away from cytotoxic activity [19]. Th17 cells in the gut play a protective role during early infection, and their depletion results in gastrointestinal inflammation and the harmful translocation of bacterial products [20]. B cells, especially tissue-like memory B cells, are overactivated in a manner similar to T cells during the chronic phase, resulting in excessive antibody production (hypergammaglobulinemia) [21]. Natural Killer (NK) cells are responsible for antiviral activity and play a major role in suppressing SIV in its natural host, but suffer from an overactivated and exhaustion-like state during the chronic phase of HIV, though this state may be reversible by *in vitro* cytokine treatment [22, 23]. Neutrophil depletion is a well-established component of HIV pathogenesis; neutrophils engage in antiviral response and may pose a protective effect against HIV but may also contribute to inflammatory pathologies [24]. Macrophages also contribute to chronic inflammation, notably HIV-associated neurocognitive disorders (HANDs) [25]. But despite prevalent foundational knowledge on lymphocytes, neutrophils, and macrophages, an understanding of the role of eosinophils and basophils in HIV is currently incomplete.

3. HIV infection and activation of eosinophils and basophils

The first step in HIV infection is the binding and entry of the virus into the host cell. The expression of surface receptors that bind to HIV on cellular targets determines viral tropism. CD4 is the primary receptor that binds to the HIV envelope (env) protein. Co-receptors and viral attachment factors also facilitate viral binding. Co-receptors include CXCR4, CCR5, and CCR3, which basophils and eosinophils express at low levels at homeostasis but can be induced upon incubation or stimulation. While the majority of peripheral granulocytes do not express CD4, subsets of neutrophils and eosinophils have low CD4 expression [26, 27]. However, granulocytes can express viral attachment receptors, which include HSPG molecules, a4b7 integrins, C-type lectins of DC-SIGN, DCIR, and mannose receptors that bind to HIV-1 gp120 [28–32]. Indeed, dendritic cells are well known to capture HIV-1 and trans-infect $CD4^+$ T cells when they form immunological synapses for antigen presentation [31]. Further, some viral attachment factors have better binding affinity to gp120. For example, DCIR has a lower binding affinity than DC-SIGN [33]. Of these HIV attachment factors, basophils express multiple factors, including DC-SIGN, CDIR, HSPG, and a4b7, while eosinophils express a4b7 [34]. Therefore, both eosinophils and basophils express HIV coreceptors and viral attachment factors necessary for HIV binding and entry (**Figure 1**).

Early in-vitro studies showed evidence that eosinophils can be directly infected with CXCR4-tropic (X4) HIV [27]. Indeed, in vitro experimental HIV-1 infection of isolated mature eosinophils [35] and bone marrow-derived $CD4^+$ eosinophil precursors cultured with IL-5 [36] indicated their potential as HIV cellular targets. HIV-1 infection in eosinophils led to their cytolysis, observed as apoptosis and necrosis *in vitro*. Productive infection in eosinophils was evidenced using HIV-1 p24 immunostaining and viral RNA in situ hybridization assays. In addition, isolated eosinophils from patients with HIV [37] showed HIV-1 sequences in 2 out of 18 patients tested, thus providing evidence of *in vivo* infection of primary eosinophils. This is further substantiated by PLWH developing hypereosinophilia concomitant with AIDS progression in the absence of ART. Even though eosinophils also express CCR5, CCR5-tropic (R5) viruses were unable to productively infect eosinophils. This was demonstrated by *Taylor et al* [38], who utilized the

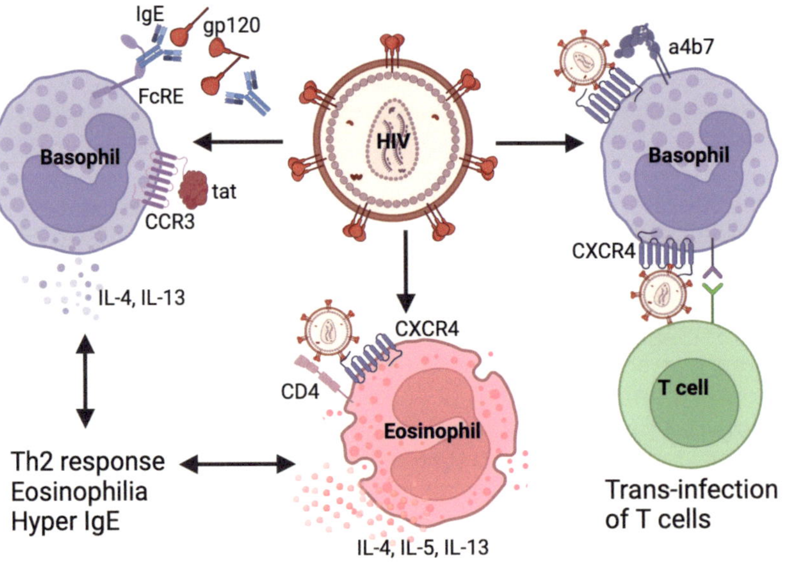

Figure 1.
HIV infection of eosinophils and basophils. Although not primary targets, eosinophils and basophils can express low levels of CD4 and HIV co-receptors (CCR, CCR5 and CXCR4). They can bind and internalize CXCR4 trophic virus particles initiating immune activation and cytokine cascade leading to Th2 type immune response. In addition, HIV gp120 and tat proteins can activate eosinophils and basophils. FcR – Fc receptor; IL – interleukin. Generated with Biorender.

eosinophilic cell line AML14.3D10 engineered to express HIV-1 coreceptors CD4, CXCR4, CCR3, and CCR5, similar to primary eosinophils for HIV-1 infection. Interestingly, viral DNA was observed only in eosinophilic cells exposed to X4 HIV-1 and not R5 HIV-1, thus indicating that R5 HIV-1 cannot enter eosinophilic cells even when appropriate coreceptors are present. Further, coreceptor blocking experiments using CXCR4 antagonist AMD3100 completely inhibited viral infection, providing proof that X4 viruses were able to infect eosinophilic cells through CXCR4 [38].

In the case of basophils, very few studies have demonstrated productive infection by HIV-1. Evidence of viral binding to basophils was provided by Jiang et al. [34] when they incubated peripheral granulocytes with viral-like particles containing HIV-Gag-GFP. Interestingly, they identified basophils to be more efficient at VLP capture than neutrophils and eosinophils. Similar to descriptions of trans-infection between dendritic cells and T cells [28, 39, 40], basophils were also capable of this phenomenon *in vitro*, which has implications for reservoir seeding in HIV infection. When HIV-1-infected basophils were co-cultured with T cells *in vitro*, they formed infectious synapses with T cells, mediating their infection upon co-culture [34]. Therefore, basophils may play important roles in HIV-1 dissemination even though they do not show productive infection.

Almost immediately following HIV-1 infection, eosinophils and basophils become activated, providing further evidence of the infection state. In their recent study of the ultrastructure of primary human eosinophils, *Melo et al* [41] were able to show in vitro eosinophil activation by HIV-1 using transmission electron microscopy. When they cultured human peripheral eosinophils with HIV-1, eosinophils showed piecemeal degranulation (PMD) whereby piece-by-piece release of secretory granule contents is achieved, allowing secretion of selective granule proteins. This was observed as granule changes combined with increased formation of tubulovesicular structures (EoSVs) in the cytoplasm of HIV-infected eosinophils. PMD in HIV-infected eosinophils could indicate an immunomodulatory function rather than effector function, because PMD allows for precise and finely tuned immune responses. Further, *Melo et al* [41] observed biogenesis of lipid droplets (LDs) leading to an increased number of giant LDs in the cytoplasm of HIV-1-infected eosinophils. LDs have been known to accumulate within host cells in response to viral infections. While LDs are considered viral assembly platforms in the case of hepatitis C [42], dengue [43] and SARS-CoV-2 [44], LDs also contain antiviral mediators and proteins that could boost antiviral defense of the host [45]. However, the role of LDs in eosinophils is currently underexplored. Overall, the substantial formation of LDs and PMD in HIV-1-infected eosinophils indicate biological processes of cellular activation post HIV infection.

Altogether, these studies clearly demonstrate binding and infection of eosinophils and basophils by HIV-1. However, there are several gaps in knowledge. What is the rate of infection of these cells and do they contribute to viral dissemination when they infiltrate tissues? Are tissue resident eosinophils at mucosal sites permissive to HIV infection and do they mediate trans-infection of HIV cellular targets at these sites. The impact of HIV infection on eosinophils and basophils also remains unclear, since they have very short half-lives in peripheral blood.

4. Antiviral immunity and inflammatory role of eosinophils and basophils in HIV infection

Eosinophils and basophils influence and maintain the immune state in a variety of disparate ways, many of which are relevant to HIV pathogenesis. One mechanism by which eosinophils defend the body against mucosal pathogens is by secretion of granule proteins: Major Basic Protein (MBP), Eosinophil Peroxidase (EPO), and arachidonic acid, which are cytotoxic and mediate inflammation. MBP promotes epithelial activation, tissue remodeling factors, the increase in smooth muscle reactivity, disrupts lipid layers and increases membrane permeability. EPO is in the eosinophil matrix and helps with the generation of reactive oxygen species (ROS) toxic to extracellular pathogens, and pro-inflammatory effects. Arachidonic acid is in the lipid bodies, which help promote acute and late hypersensitivity responses [46]. Basophils have pre-formed histamine and leukotrienes in their granules, which are potent bronchoconstrictors that cause smooth muscle contraction and increase vascular permeability. In addition, both eosinophils and basophils have several inflammatory cytokines and chemokines in their granules, which are released upon infection.

The strongest indicators of eosinophil and basophil involvement in HIV immunopathogenesis are the frequent observations of eosinophilia, elevated eosinophilic cationic protein and hyper IgE levels that have been commonly described in PLWH, even in the absence of parasitic load [47, 48]. Indeed, eosinophilia and IgE levels were important clinical features of HIV infection prior to ART therapy. Further, basophils were largely responsible for the effect of HIV on increased systemic histamine [49]. As early as 1991, it was shown that peripheral leukocytes challenged with HIV antigen led to an IgE-dependent increase in histamine production by basophils in PLWH but not healthy controls [50]. Furthermore, greater histamine production by basophils from PLWH corresponded to lower CD4+ T cell counts [50]. Histamine leads to broad inflammation as well as skewing of Th1 CD4 T cells into Th2 cells, which in conjunction with B-cell Activating Factor (BAFF), IL-4, and IL-6 produced by basophils might contribute to B cell overactivation and hypergammaglobulinemia in HIV [49]. Basophil IL-4 production also polarizes macrophages into the anti-inflammatory M2 state known to increase as chronic infection progresses. This is facilitated by HIV gp120 which acts as a superantigen interacting with the Vh3 region of IgE, activating basophils and mast cells [51]. The HIV Tat protein also acts as a chemoattractant for basophils by targeting the CCR3 receptor and simultaneously driving increased CCR3 expression on these cells, thereby amplifying their recruitment and activation [52, 53]. Based on these studies and observations, Becker, in 2004 [54, 55], hypothesized that HIV gp120 mimics allergens by binding to IgE and activated basophils, mast cells, and eosinophils, which in turn promote IL-4 secretion and drive a Th2-type immune response rather than a Th1 response. This led to the proposition that the HIV immune response resembles an allergic reaction. However, eosinophilia was predominantly associated with untreated HIV, and low CD4+ T cell counts and typically resolves following initiation of ART. Overall, eosinophilia and hypergammaglobulinemia are primarily due to HIV mediated shift to Th2 type of immune response characterized by increased production of IL-4, IL5 and IL-13 cytokines, which in turn favor development, recruitment and survival of eosinophils and basophils. Nonetheless, further studies are needed to determine the clinical significance of eosinophils and basophils in HIV acquisition and disease progression, since excessive activation of these cells can result in inflammatory conditions.

In PLWH treated with ART, eosinophilia and eosinophilic manifestations still occur in certain instances. For example, elevated eosinophils were associated with hypertension in ART-treated PLWH but not in HIV negative individuals [56]. Similarly, cases of eosinophilic folliculitis and dermatosis, acute eosinophilic myocarditis, and eosinophilic meningitis have been described in PLWH [57, 58] that provide evidence of the inflammatory role of eosinophils in HIV infection. Interestingly, in a study [59] that comparing three groups of PLWH undergoing ART- treatment failures (patients in whom ART fails to suppress viral replication), treatment responders (patients with successful viral suppression and CD4+ T cell restoration), and virologic non-responders (those for whom ART does suppress virus but restores CD4+ T cells), high levels of IL-5, eosinophil frequency, and T-regs were observed only in virologic non-responders. Typically, virologic failure occurs in patients with low CD4+ T cell counts at ART initiation reflecting the critical roles immune cells play in controlling viral replication. In the case of virologic non-responders, virologic failure, that is unsuppressed viremia occurs even though immune recovery/increased CD4+ T cell counts after ART initiation indicates a decoupling of viral control and immune reconstitution. The increased IL-5 and eosinophilia in this group could suggest Th2 response, potentially leading to unsuccessful viral suppression. These findings indicate complex immunological milieu in HIV infection and underscore the need to better understand granulocyte biology in HIV infection. In addition, eosinophil-mediated inflammatory processes could drive non-AIDS comorbidities even in virus-suppressed PLWH and necessitates more studies exploring the role of eosinophils in chronic viral inflammation.

The degree to which basophils and eosinophils function as antigen-presenting cells (APCs) is an ongoing topic in granulocyte research, and the role of this axis of immune activity in HIV/AIDS is poorly understood [60]. At best, eosinophils and basophils can work as weak APCs. As mentioned previously, basophils can transfer HIV virus to CD4+ T cells after forming immunological synapses, though the nature of these synapses and whether they facilitate antigen presentation is not completely clear [34]. Eosinophils express MHCII molecules and can present parasite antigen to T cells, leading to Th2 polarization [60]. While processing and presentation of viral antigens by eosinophils have not yet been reported, bone marrow-derived eosinophils were found to upregulate antigen-presenting molecules including MHCI and CD86 after exposure to Influenza A virus [61]. Therefore, it is possible that eosinophils and basophils can act as APCs under certain conditions.

Of all the granulocyte cells, neutrophils have been more studied in HIV infection. Since eosinophils and basophils share a common myeloid progenitor with neutrophils and perform similar functions, it is reasonable to hypothesize overlapping roles in antiviral defense. Neutrophils are capable of forming inflammatory neutrophil extracellular traps (NETS), which can trap and neutralize pathogens through a process called NETosis. These NETS have been described to have protective roles in HIV-1 infection. Stimulation of human genital neutrophils with HIV VLPS *in vitro* resulted in NET release and HIV-VLP entrapment within minutes of viral exposure [62]. NETS can also modulate the functioning of the HIV-1 target cell. When *in vitro* HIV-1-infected macrophages were exposed to NETs, restriction of HIV-1 replication was observed [63]. Since eosinophils and basophils can similarly deploy extracellular traps through eosinophil EETs and basophil BETs, respectively, they may capture virions, neutralize viral spread, and recruit immune effectors to the site of infection.

Eosinophils produce several antiviral compounds such as guanylate binding proteins (GBPs), specialized pro-resolving mediators (SPMs), eosinophil cationic protein (ECP), and eosinophil-derived neurotoxin (EDN), and are recognized as important contributors to antiviral immunity against respiratory syncytial virus (RSV) and influenza A virus in the lungs [61, 64]. But their ability to exert antiviral effects in the context of HIV has not been studied so far [65]. Furthermore, eosinophils isolated from rhesus macaque infected with Simian-Human Immunodeficiency Virus (SHIV) displayed functional differences from those of naïve animals, with *ex vivo* stimulation with lipopolysaccharide eliciting increased production of IL-8, a neutrophil chemoattractant implicated in chronic HIV inflammation -in comparison to eosinophils from uninfected controls [66]. These observations suggest that lentiviral infection may reprogram eosinophil functional responses toward roles that perpetuate immune activation. Understanding whether this functional plasticity contributes to HIV persistence or pathogenesis could uncover novel targets for modulating the inflammatory milieu in PLWH.

5. Tissue eosinophils and basophils in HIV infection

There are several organs where eosinophils are found under homeostatic conditions, unlike basophils, which are rarely present in peripheral tissues during homeostasis. Eosinophils are enriched in the gut, thymus, uterus, and mammary gland where they can play important homeostatic and regulatory functions. For example, at homeostasis, the gastrointestinal tract harbors the largest population of tissue resident eosinophils which have specific characteristics such as altered phenotype, signs of degranulation and prolonged survival and are important for gut homeostasis [67, 68]. They are recruited to the gut during late gestation and early life independent of the microbiota [69]. During normal physiological conditions, gut-residing eosinophils are involved in immuno-regulation, maintenance of other immune cell populations, and the protection of the mucosal barrier [69]. Gut-residing eosinophils interaction with immune cells is important to providing immunity to the microbiota, which inhabits the lumen of the gut [69] and they promote tissue repair and promote barrier function during homeostasis and inflammation. In a mouse model of dextran sodium sulfate (DSS) induced colitis, reduced intestinal pathology was observed via eosinophil production of protective lipid mediator protectin D1 which dampened inflammatory mediators [70]. Further, in the absence of eosinophils, neutrophils are compensatory increased in the gut which in turn lead to colitis [70]. They maintain microbial homeostasis, at least in part, due to their role in retaining IgA- producing plasma cells in Peyer's patches [71]. Interestingly, even in the absence of inflammation, high-fat diet feeding in mice leads to intestinal eosinophil depletion which in turn is associated with intestinal permeability [72]. Given the importance of eosinophils in the intestine, studies assessing their role in HIV immunity have been lacking. While homeostatic eosinophils have not been studied in relation to HIV, their role in polarizing TH17 cells into regulatory T cells could inform immune evasion and reservoir perpetuation in the mucosa [73].

Recent studies by our group using an NHP model of HIV infection, showed significant reduction in the frequency of circulating basophils in SHIV-infected rhesus macaques [74]. However, it is not clear if this was due to HIV-mediated apoptosis of these cells or infiltration of basophils into tissues, since basophils have been known to infiltrate tissues during parasitic infection [75, 76]. In the same study, we characterized the frequencies of neutrophils, eosinophils, and basophils in different tissues including spleen, axillary lymph nodes, liver, jejunum, colorectal and vaginal tissues. In chronic SHIV-infected rhesus macaques, reduced eosinophil frequencies were observed in the jejunum and vaginal tissues compared to naïve animals, indicating that HIV may mediate depletion of eosinophils in mucosa tissues. Interestingly, colorectal biopsy tissues showed elevated eosinophil frequencies, which could indicate increased infiltration of these granulocytes in mucosal sites of infection. No differences were observed in frequencies of tissue basophils. There are several gaps in knowledge - Are tissue eosinophils and basophils susceptible to HIV? Are jejunal eosinophils important antiviral immune effectors and does their depletion in HIV infection impact gut permeability, which is a hallmark sequela of HIV infection. Are tissue eosinophils inflammatory in HIV infection, leading to pathologic inflammation of the gut and mucosal tissues, aggravating HIV disease? Pathologic eosinophil infiltration of the gut can lead to chronic inflammatory disorder called eosinophilic gastrointestinal disorder (EGID) and is associated with food allergy triggers [77]. Overall, more studies are needed to elucidate the role of tissue eosinophils and basophils in HIV infection.

6. Therapeutic/vaccine implications of eosinophils and basophils

In the context of HIV infection, the development of vaccines and therapeutics remain a crucial priority. While ART is highly effective at suppressing viral replication and preventing disease progression, ART alone is insufficient to eradicate the virus, since HIV establishes latent reservoirs despite long term treatment. Therefore, innovative strategies are urgently needed to either eliminate latent infection or achieve durable immune control in the absence of ART. Eosinophils and basophils represent underexplored allies in antiviral immunity, capable of amplifying protective responses. As first responders of immunity during infections, these cell subsets may influence disease progression and vaccine efficacy due to their myriad effector functions: interactions with T cells and other immune cells, antigen presentation, cytokine networks, tissue remodeling, and regulatory roles. Their roles in trained immunity and tissue resident responses are also emerging areas with therapeutic relevance. However, excessive or unchecked activation could drive pathological inflammation, undermining host defense. Therefore, in this section, we will outline vaccine and therapeutic strategies that harness the beneficial effector functions of these subsets as well as approaches aimed at selectively depleting these cells when necessary (**Figure 2**).

Eosinophils and basophils express a repertoire of Fc receptors either at homeostasis or post-stimulation. These include activating FcgRs (CD64 and CD32), high-affinity IgE receptor (FceRI), and mucosal relevant IgA binding receptor (CD89). This positions them as key effector cells in antibody-mediated immunity. Through Fc-antibody interactions, these cells can engage in antibody-based effector functions, which include cytotoxicity, phagocytosis, release of cytokines, chemokines, and antiviral mediators already present in their granules. For HIV infection, anti-HIV-1 broadly neutralizing antibodies are effective in preventing infection, lowering viremia, and maintaining viral suppression as standalone maintenance treatments or as an adjunct to ART [78–81]. FcR engagement on eosinophils and basophils may enhance viral clearance through direct effector functions as seen in other FcR-bearing effector cells such as neutrophils, NK cells, and monocytes.

To utilize the FcR and extracellular trap-mediated functions of eosinophils and basophils and to maximize the efficacy of antibody-based therapeutics, enhancing the frequency, activation, and trafficking of these subsets into mucosal sites of HIV infection represents an important strategy. Adjuvants such as granulocyte-macrophage colony-stimulating factor (GM-CSF) can rapidly mobilize granulocytes from bone marrow and enhance their functional antibody-mediated functions, thereby improving host defenses against pathogens [82–84]. GM-CSF in combination with anti-HIV-1bNAbs may provide an effective HIV therapeutic strategy. Indeed, preclinical studies

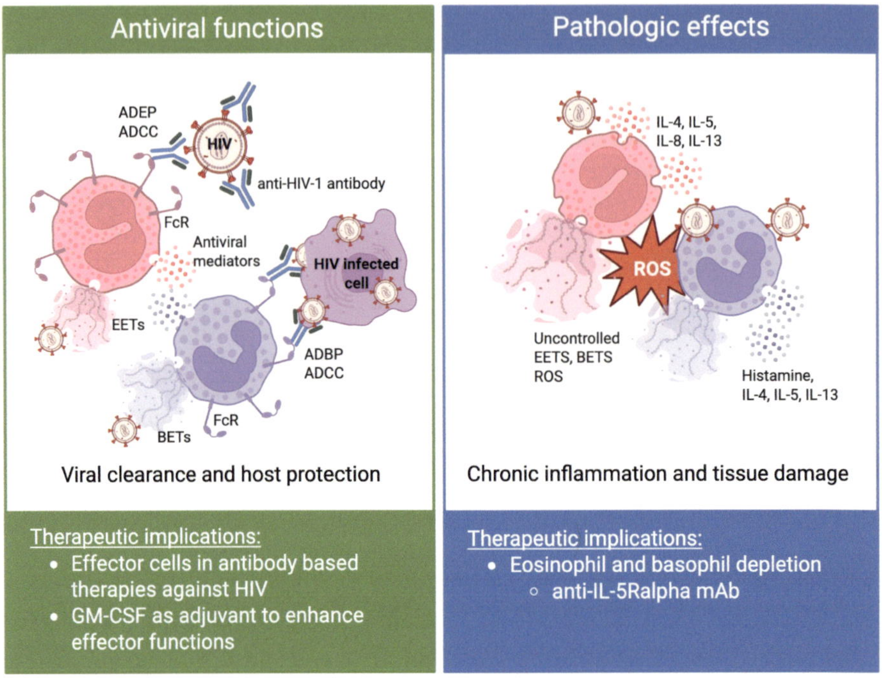

Figure 2.
Dual roles of eosinophils and basophils in lentiviral infection. Eosinophils and basophils can contribute to HIV clearance through extracellular trap generation, secretion of antiviral mediators (which includes eosinophilic cationic protein, guanylate-binding proteins, antiviral cytokines) and antibody mediated functions. However, persistent activation of eosinophils and basophils can drive excessive release of pro-inflammatory mediators and cytotoxic granule proteins contributing to tissue damage, fibrosis and immune dysregulation. Based on these dual roles, interventions may aim to enhance their antiviral and immunoregulatory functions while curbing their pathogenic inflammatory effects. ADCC - antibody dependent cell cytotoxicity; ADBP - antibody dependent basophil phagocytosis; ADEP - antibody dependent eosinophil phagocytosis; BETs - basophil extracellular traps; EETs - eosinophil extracellular traps; FcR – Fc receptor; IL – interleukin; mAb – monoclonal antibody; ROS – reactive oxygen species. Generated with Biorender.

using a DNA vaccine against HIV Gag protein with a GM-CSF plasmid as an adjuvant were tested in mice and rhesus macaques and were found to enhance HIV-specific antibody and T cell responses [85]. However, this study did not evaluate the impact of this DNA vaccine and GM-CSF on granulocytes. Other studies in PLWH for treatment of HIV associated conditions such as Kaposi sarcoma, cytomegalovirus retinitis, and non-Hodgkin lymphoma have utilized GM-CSF [86–89]. Currently, GM-CSF is being evaluated as an adjuvant for Hepatitis B vaccination in PLWH (NCT00272493).

Conversely, therapeutics aimed at limiting eosinophil and basophil activity may improve inflammation caused by HIV. The anti-IL5 Rα monoclonal antibody Benralizumab has been shown in several clinical trials to deplete eosinophils and limit the severity of eosinophilic esophagitis [90], a comorbidity of HIV [91]. Benralizumab can be employed to alleviate this pathology in PLWH and could potentially be expanded to treat other pathologies related to HIV-induced eosinophilia. Methods for basophil depletion are less developed, but anti-CD200R3 monoclonal antibody shows promise a selective basophil-depletion therapy, decreasing IgE-mediated anaphylaxis in a mouse study [92]. The effect of basophil depletion in HIV beyond a decrease in circulating histamines is uncertain, but given the diversity of basophil function, such a therapy may regulate other pathways of immune overactivation.

It is also important to consider that the granulocyte subtypes are still distinct and may contribute to antiviral defense through different pathways while designing vaccines/adjuvants to induce innate granulocytes. This was evidenced in a clinical trial study evaluating an HIV-1 gp41 membrane-proximal external region (MPER)-peptide liposome immunogen in HIV-1 seronegative individuals [93]. Interestingly, neutrophils responded robustly to MPER-peptide-liposomes and even anti-polyethylene glycol antibodies by elevating CD63 expression, a sign of their degranulation, whereas not basophils did not show any degranulation in response to the same stimuli. This finding underscores the cell type specificity of innate immune activation by vaccine components and suggests that targeting eosinophils and basophils may require distinct adjuvant or immunogen designs to effectively engage their antiviral functions.

7. Conclusion

In summary, eosinophils and basophils represent important but understudied components of the immune landscape in HIV infection. Eosinophilia and hyper IgE levels are evidence of the activation of these granulocytic subsets in HIV infection and indicate a potential role in HIV immunopathogenesis that extends beyond their traditional functions in allergy and parasitic defense. While much remains to be understood regarding their roles in viral control and/or dissemination, immune activation, and tissue inflammation, these granulocytes offer promising avenues as newer therapeutic and vaccine strategies aimed at modulating innate immunity are developed. Future research focused on defining their interactions with antibody-based therapies, specific adjuvants and activation mechanisms, and their impact on the chronic inflammatory milieu may unlock novel opportunities to enhance immune control and improve outcomes for PLWH.

Acknowledgements

The authors want to thank Griffin Woolley for helpful comments on the chapter. Work described in this chapter was supported in part by NIH grant R21AI172030 to C.M.

Conflict of interest

The authors declare no conflict of interest.

Author details

Cordelia Manickam[1,2], Andrew Hudson[1,2] and R. Keith Reeves[1,2]*

1 Division of Innate and Comparative Immunology, Center for Human Systems Immunology, Duke University School of Medicine, Durham, North Carolina, USA

2 Department of Surgery, Duke University School of Medicine, Durham, North Carolina, USA

*Address all correspondence to: keith.reeves@duke.edu

References

[1] De Cock KM, Jaffe HW, Curran JW. Reflections on 30 years of AIDS. Emerging Infectious Diseases. 2011;**17**(6):1044-1048

[2] Meissner ME, Talledge N, Mansky LM. Molecular biology and diversification of human retroviruses. Frontiers in Virology. 2022;**2**:872599

[3] Sharp PM, Hahn BH. Origins of HIV and the AIDS pandemic. Cold Spring Harbor Perspectives in Medicine. 2011;**1**(1):a006841

[4] Chen Y, Li AD, Yang Y, Lu J, Xu Y, Ji X, et al. Global, regional and national burden of HIV/AIDS among individuals aged 15-79 from 1990 to 2021. AIDS Research and Therapy. 2025;**22**(1):51

[5] Shaw GM, Hunter E. HIV transmission. Cold Spring Harbor Perspectives in Medicine. 2012;**2**(11):a006965

[6] Tseng A, Seet J, Phillips EJ. The evolution of three decades of antiretroviral therapy: Challenges, triumphs and the promise of the future. British Journal of Clinical Pharmacology. 2015;**79**(2):182-194

[7] HIV/AIDS Factsheet [Press Release]. United Nations Office for the Coordination of Humanitarian Affairs. UNAIDS; 2023. Available from: https://www.unaids.org/sites/default/files/2025-07/2025_Global_HIV_Factsheet_en.pdf

[8] Nkolola JP, Barouch DH. Prophylactic HIV-1 vaccine trials: Past, present, and future. Lancet HIV. 2024;**11**(2):e117-ee24

[9] Threats M, Brawner BM, Montgomery TM, Abrams J, Jemmott LS, Crouch PC, et al. A review of recent HIV prevention interventions and future considerations for nursing science. The Journal of the Association of Nurses in AIDS Care. 2021;**32**(3):373-391

[10] Sabin CA. Do people with HIV infection have a normal life expectancy in the era of combination antiretroviral therapy? BMC Medicine. 2013;**11**:251

[11] Weichseldorfer M, Reitz M, Latinovic OS. Past HIV-1 medications and the current status of combined antiretroviral therapy options for HIV-1 patients. Pharmaceutics. 2021;**13**(11):1798

[12] Banga R, Perreau M. The multifaceted nature of HIV tissue reservoirs. Current Opinion in HIV and AIDS. 2024;**19**(3):116-123

[13] Apetroaei MM, Velescu B, Nedea MII, Dinu-Pîrvu CE, Drăgănescu D, Fâcă AI, et al. The phenomenon of antiretroviral drug resistance in the context of human immunodeficiency virus treatment: Dynamic and ever evolving subject matter. Biomedicine. 2024;**12**(4):915

[14] Kim Y, Anderson JL, Lewin SR. Getting the "kill" into "shock and kill": Strategies to eliminate latent HIV. Cell Host & Microbe. 2018;**23**(1):14-26

[15] Desai M, Field N, Grant R, McCormack S. Recent advances in pre-exposure prophylaxis for HIV. BMJ. 2017;**359**:j5011

[16] Cao W, Mehraj V, Kaufmann DE, Li T, Routy JP. Elevation and persistence of CD8 T-cells in HIV infection: The Achilles heel in the ART era. Journal of the International AIDS Society. 2016;**19**(1):20697

[17] Fenwick C, Joo V, Jacquier P, Noto A, Banga R, Perreau M, et al. T-cell exhaustion in HIV infection. Immunological Reviews. 2019;**292**(1):149-163

[18] Collins DR, Gaiha GD, Walker BD. CD8(+) T cells in HIV control, cure and prevention. Nature Reviews. Immunology. 2020;**20**(8):471-482

[19] Hokello J, Tyagi K, Owor RO, Sharma AL, Bhushan A, Daniel R, et al. New insights into HIV life cycle, Th1/Th2 shift during HIV infection and preferential virus infection of Th2 cells: Implications of early HIV treatment initiation and care. Life (Basel). 2024;**14**(1):104

[20] Elhed A, Unutmaz D. Th17 cells and HIV infection. Current Opinion in HIV and AIDS. 2010;**5**(2):146-150

[21] Moir S, Fauci AS. B-cell exhaustion in HIV infection: The role of immune activation. Current Opinion in HIV and AIDS. 2014;**9**(5):472-477

[22] Moreno-Cubero E, Alrubayyi A, Balint S, Ogbe A, Gill US, Matthews R, et al. IL-15 reprogramming compensates for NK cell mitochondrial dysfunction in HIV-1 infection. JCI Insight. 2024;**9**(4):e173099

[23] Schafer JL, Müller-Trutwin MC, Reeves RK. NK cell exhaustion: Bad news for chronic disease? Oncotarget. 2015;**6**:21797-21798

[24] Madzime M, Rossouw TM, Theron AJ, Anderson R, Steel HC. Interactions of HIV and antiretroviral therapy with neutrophils and platelets. Frontiers in Immunology. 2021;**12**:634386

[25] Kruize Z, Kootstra NA. The role of macrophages in HIV-1 persistence and pathogenesis. Frontiers in Microbiology. 2019;**10**:2828

[26] Biswas P, Mantelli B, Sica A, Malnati M, Panzeri C, Saccani A, et al. Expression of CD4 on human peripheral blood neutrophils. Blood. 2003;**101**(11):4452-4456

[27] Lucey DR, Dorsky DI, Nicholson-Weller A, Weller PF. Human eosinophils express CD4 protein and bind human immunodeficiency virus 1 gp120. The Journal of Experimental Medicine. 1989;**169**(1):327-332

[28] Ahmed Z, Kawamura T, Shimada S, Piguet V. The role of human dendritic cells in HIV-1 infection. The Journal of Investigative Dermatology. 2015;**135**(5):1225-1233

[29] Vives RR, Imberty A, Sattentau QJ, Lortat-Jacob H. Heparan sulfate targets the HIV-1 envelope glycoprotein gp120 coreceptor binding site. The Journal of Biological Chemistry. 2005;**280**(22):21353-21357

[30] Arthos J, Cicala C, Martinelli E, Macleod K, Van Ryk D, Wei D, et al. HIV-1 envelope protein binds to and signals through integrin alpha4beta7, the gut mucosal homing receptor for peripheral T cells. Nature Immunology. 2008;**9**(3):301-309

[31] Wu L, KewalRamani VN. Dendritic-cell interactions with HIV: Infection and viral dissemination. Nature Reviews. Immunology. 2006;**6**(11):859-868

[32] Wilen CB, Tilton JC, Doms RW. HIV: Cell binding and entry. Cold Spring Harbor Perspectives in Medicine. 2012;**2**(8):a006866

[33] Jin W, Li C, Du T, Hu K, Huang X, Hu Q. DC-SIGN plays a stronger role than DCIR in mediating HIV-1 capture and transfer. Virology. 2014;**458-459**:83-92

[34] Jiang AP, Jiang JF, Guo MG, Jin YM, Li YY, Wang JH. Human blood-circulating basophils capture HIV-1 and mediate viral trans-infection of CD4+ T cells. Journal of Virology. 2015;**89**(15):8050-8062

[35] Weller PF, Marshall WL, Lucey DR, Rand TH, Dvorak AM, Finberg RW. Infection, apoptosis, and killing of mature human eosinophils by human immunodeficiency virus-1. American Journal of Respiratory Cell and Molecular Biology. 1995;**13**(5):610-620

[36] Freedman AR, Gibson FM, Fleming SC, Spry CJ, Griffin GE. Human immunodeficiency virus infection of eosinophils in human bone marrow cultures. The Journal of Experimental Medicine. 1991;**174**(6):1661-1664

[37] Conway B, Baskar P, Bechtel LJ, Kaplan JC, Hirsch MS, Schooley RT, et al. Eosinophils as host cells for HIV-1. Archives of Virology. 1992;**127**(1-4):373-377

[38] Taylor RJ, Schols D, Wooley DP. Restricted entry of R5 HIV type 1 strains into eosinophilic cells. AIDS Research and Human Retroviruses. 2004;**20**(11):1244-1253

[39] Martin N, Sattentau Q. Cell-to-cell HIV-1 spread and its implications for immune evasion. Current Opinion in HIV and AIDS. 2009;**4**(2):143-149

[40] Shen R, Kappes JC, Smythies LE, Richter HE, Novak L, Smith PD. Vaginal myeloid dendritic cells transmit founder HIV-1. Journal of Virology. 2014;**88**(13):7683-7688

[41] Melo RCN, Silva TP. Eosinophil activation during immune responses: An ultrastructural view with an emphasis on viral diseases. Journal of Leukocyte Biology. 2024;**116**(2):321-334

[42] Roingeard P, Hourioux C. Hepatitis C virus core protein, lipid droplets and steatosis. Journal of Viral Hepatitis. 2008;**15**(3):157-164

[43] Samsa MM, Mondotte JA, Iglesias NG, Assuncao-Miranda I, Barbosa-Lima G, Da Poian AT, et al. Dengue virus capsid protein usurps lipid droplets for viral particle formation. PLoS Pathogens. 2009;**5**(10):e1000632

[44] Dias SSG, Soares VC, Ferreira AC, Sacramento CQ, Fintelman-Rodrigues N, Temerozo JR, et al. Lipid droplets fuel SARS-CoV-2 replication and production of inflammatory mediators. PLoS Pathogens. 2020;**16**(12):e1009127

[45] Monson EA, Trenerry AM, Laws JL, Mackenzie JM, Helbig KJ. Lipid droplets and lipid mediators in viral infection and immunity. FEMS Microbiology Reviews. 2021;**45**(4):fuaa066

[46] Ramirez GA, Yacoub MR, Ripa M, Mannina D, Cariddi A, Saporiti N, et al. Eosinophils from physiology to disease: A comprehensive review. BioMed Research International. 2018;**2018**:9095275

[47] Cohen AJ, Steigbigel RT. Eosinophilia in patients infected with human immunodeficiency virus. The Journal of Infectious Diseases. 1996;**174**(3):615-618

[48] Al Mohajer M, Villarreal-Williams E, Andrade RA, Giordano TP, Serpa JA. Eosinophilia and associated factors in a large cohort of patients infected with human immunodeficiency virus. Southern Medical Journal. 2014;**107**(9):554-558

[49] Shah H, Eisenbarth S, Tormey CA, Siddon AJ. Behind the scenes with basophils: An emerging therapeutic target. Immunotherapy Advances. 2021;**1**(1):ltab008

[50] Pedersen M, Nielsen CM, Permin H. HIV antigen-induced release of histamine from basophils from HIV infected patients. Mechanism and relation to disease progression and immunodeficiency. Allergy. 1991;**46**(3):206-212

[51] Florio G, Petraroli A, Patella V, Triggiani M, Marone G. The immunoglobulin superantigen-binding site of HIV-1 gp120 activates human basophils. AIDS. 2000;**14**(8):931-938

[52] Albini A, Ferrini S, Benelli R, Sforzini S, Giunciuglio D, Aluigi MG, et al. HIV-1 Tat protein mimicry of chemokines. Proceedings of the National Academy of Sciences of the United States of America. 1998;**95**(22):13153-13158

[53] de Paulis A, De Palma R, Di Gioia L, Carfora M, Prevete N, Tosi G, et al. Tat protein is an HIV-1-encoded beta-chemokine homolog that promotes migration and up-regulates CCR3 expression on human Fc epsilon RI+ cells. Journal of Immunology. 2000;**165**(12):7171-7179

[54] Becker Y. A point of view: HIV-1/AIDS is an allergy but CpG ODN treatments may inhibit virus replication and reactivate the adaptive immunity–hypothesis and implications. Virus Genes. 2005;**30**(1):127-131

[55] Becker Y. HIV-1 induced AIDS is an allergy and the allergen is the shed gp120–A review, hypothesis, and implications. Virus Genes. 2004;**28**(3):319-331

[56] Masenga SK, Elijovich F, Hamooya BM, Nzala S, Kwenda G, Heimburger DC, et al. Elevated eosinophils as a feature of inflammation associated with hypertension in virally suppressed people living with HIV. Journal of the American Heart Association. 2020;**9**(4):e011450

[57] Thawabi M, Habib M, Shaaban H, Shamoon F. Acute eosinophilic myocarditis and hyper IgE in HIV infection: A case report. North American Journal of Medical Sciences. 2014;**6**(7):338-341

[58] de Almeida SM, de Souza CV, Pletsch L, Kovaliuk SK, Hummelgen A Jr, Piseta VV, et al. Diagnostic importance of eosinophilic meningitis in HIV-positive and HIV-negative patients. Journal of Neurovirology. 2019;**25**(3):331-341

[59] Shete A, Kurle S, Dhayarkar S, Patil A, Kulkarni S, Ghate M, et al. High IL-5 levels possibly contributing to HIV viremia in virologic non-responders at one year after initiation of anti-retroviral therapy. Microbial Pathogenesis. 2020;**143**:104117

[60] Lin A, Loré K. Granulocytes: New members of the antigen-presenting cell family. Frontiers in Immunology. 2017;**8**:1781

[61] Samarasinghe AE, Melo RC, Duan S, LeMessurier KS, Liedmann S, Surman SL, et al. Eosinophils promote antiviral immunity in mice infected with influenza a virus. Journal of Immunology. 2017;**198**(8):3214-3226

[62] Barr FD, Ochsenbauer C, Wira CR, Rodriguez-Garcia M. Neutrophil extracellular traps prevent HIV infection in the female genital tract. Mucosal Immunology. 2018;**11**(5):1420-1428

[63] Mojoli A, Goncalves BS, Temerozo JR, Cister-Alves B, Geddes V, Herlinger A, et al. Neutrophil extracellular traps from healthy donors and HIV-1-infected individuals restrict HIV-1 production in macrophages. Scientific Reports. 2020;**10**(1):19603

[64] Phipps S, Lam CE, Mahalingam S, Newhouse M, Ramirez R, Rosenberg HF, et al. Eosinophils contribute to innate antiviral immunity and promote clearance of respiratory syncytial virus. Blood. 2007;**110**(5):1578-1586

[65] Sasaki H, Miyata J, Kawana A, Fukunaga K. Antiviral roles of eosinophils in asthma and respiratory viral infection. Frontiers in Allergy. 2025;**6**:1548338

[66] Jones R, Afifi A, Reeves RK, Manickam C. Functional reprogramming of peripheral eosinophils in lentivirus-infected rhesus macaques. AIDS Research and Human Retroviruses. 2025;**41**(8):411-413

[67] Mishra A, Hogan SP, Lee JJ, Foster PS, Rothenberg ME. Fundamental signals that regulate eosinophil homing to the gastrointestinal tract. The Journal of Clinical Investigation. 1999;**103**(12):1719-1727

[68] Gurtner A, Gonzalez-Perez I, Arnold IC. Intestinal eosinophils, homeostasis and response to bacterial intrusion. Seminars in Immunopathology. 2021;**43**(3):295-306

[69] Loktionov A. Eosinophils in the gastrointestinal tract and their role in the pathogenesis of major colorectal disorders. World Journal of Gastroenterology. 2019;**25**(27):3503-3526

[70] Masterson JC, McNamee EN, Fillon SA, Hosford L, Harris R, Fernando SD, et al. Eosinophil-mediated signalling attenuates inflammatory responses in experimental colitis. Gut. 2015;**64**(8):1236-1247

[71] Chu VT, Beller A, Rausch S, Strandmark J, Zanker M, Arbach O, et al. Eosinophils promote generation and maintenance of immunoglobulin-A-expressing plasma cells and contribute to gut immune homeostasis. Immunity. 2014;**40**(4):582-593

[72] Johnson AM, Costanzo A, Gareau MG, Armando AM, Quehenberger O, Jameson JM, et al. High fat diet causes depletion of intestinal eosinophils associated with intestinal permeability. PLoS One. 2015;**10**(4):e0122195

[73] Marichal T, Mesnil C, Bureau F. Homeostatic eosinophils: Characteristics and functions. Frontiers in Medicine (Lausanne). 2017;**4**:101

[74] Jones R, Manickam C, Ram DR, Kroll K, Hueber B, Woolley G, et al. Systemic and mucosal mobilization of granulocyte subsets during lentiviral infection. Immunology. 2021;**164**(2):348-357

[75] de Paulis A, Prevete N, Fiorentino I, Walls AF, Curto M, Petraroli A, et al. Basophils infiltrate human gastric mucosa at sites of helicobacter pylori infection, and exhibit chemotaxis in response to *H. pylori*-derived peptide Hp(2-20). Journal of Immunology. 2004;**172**(12):7734-7743

[76] Schroeder JT. Basophils: Emerging roles in the pathogenesis of allergic disease. Immunological Reviews. 2011;**242**(1):144-160

[77] Gonsalves N. Eosinophilic gastrointestinal disorders. Clinical Reviews in Allergy and Immunology. 2019;**57**(2):272-285

[78] Caskey M. Broadly neutralizing antibodies for the treatment and prevention of HIV infection. Current Opinion in HIV and AIDS. 2020;**15**(1):49-55

[79] Mendoza P, Gruell H, Nogueira L, Pai JA, Butler AL, Millard K, et al. Combination therapy with anti-HIV-1 antibodies maintains viral suppression. Nature. 2018;**561**(7724):479-484

[80] Corey L, Gilbert PB, Juraska M, Montefiori DC, Morris L, Karuna ST, et al. Two randomized trials of neutralizing antibodies to prevent HIV-1 acquisition. The New England Journal of Medicine. 2021;**384**(11):1003-1014

[81] Gaebler C, Nogueira L, Stoffel E, Oliveira TY, Breton G, Millard KG, et al. Prolonged viral suppression with anti-HIV-1 antibody therapy. Nature. 2022;**606**(7913):368-374

[82] Spiekermann K, Roesler J, Emmendoerffer A, Elsner J, Welte K. Functional features of neutrophils induced by G-CSF and GM-CSF treatment: Differential effects and clinical implications. Leukemia. 1997;**11**(4):466-478

[83] Barreda DR, Hanington PC, Belosevic M. Regulation of myeloid development and function by colony stimulating factors. Developmental and Comparative Immunology. 2004;**28**(5):509-554

[84] Ushach I, Zlotnik A. Biological role of granulocyte macrophage colony-stimulating factor (GM-CSF) and macrophage colony-stimulating factor (M-CSF) on cells of the myeloid lineage. Journal of Leukocyte Biology. 2016;**100**(3):481-489

[85] Song R, Liu S, Adams RJ, Leong KW. Enhancing efficacy of HIV gag DNA vaccine by local delivery of GM-CSF in murine and macaque models. Journal of Interferon & Cytokine Research. 2006;**26**(6):380-389

[86] Hardy WD. Combined ganciclovir and recombinant human granulocyte-macrophage colony-stimulating factor in the treatment of cytomegalovirus retinitis in AIDS patients. Journal of Acquired Immune Deficiency Syndromes (1988). 1991;**4**(Suppl. 1):S22-S28

[87] Kaplan LD, Kahn JO, Crowe S, Northfelt D, Neville P, Grossberg H, et al. Clinical and virologic effects of recombinant human granulocyte-macrophage colony-stimulating factor in patients receiving chemotherapy for human immunodeficiency virus-associated non-Hodgkin's lymphoma: Results of a randomized trial. Journal of Clinical Oncology. 1991;**9**(6):929-940

[88] Gill PS, Mitsuyasu RT, Montgomery T, Huang J, Cabriales S, Testa M, et al. AIDS clinical trials group study 094: A phase I/II trial of ABV chemotherapy with zidovudine and recombinant human GM-CSF in AIDS-related Kaposi's sarcoma. The Cancer Journal from Scientific American. 1997;**3**(5):278-283

[89] Deresinski SC. Granulocyte-macrophage colony-stimulating factor: Potential therapeutic, immunological and antiretroviral effects in HIV infection. AIDS. 1999;**13**(6):633-643

[90] Rothenberg ME, Dellon ES, Collins MH, Bredenoord AJ, Hirano I, Peterson KA, et al. Eosinophil depletion with Benralizumab for eosinophilic esophagitis. The New England Journal of Medicine. 2024;**390**(24):2252-2263

[91] Asfari MM, Kendrick K, Sarmini MT, Uy P, Vega KJ. Association of eosinophilic esophagitis and human immunodeficiency virus. Digestive Diseases and Sciences. 2021;**66**(8):2669-2673

[92] Nakamura T, Fukaya T, Uto T, Takagi H, Arimura K, Tono T, et al. Selective depletion of basophils ameliorates immunoglobulin E-mediated anaphylaxis. Biochemistry and Biophysics Reports. 2017;**9**:29-35

[93] Erdmann NB, Williams WB, Walsh SR, Grunenberg N, Edlefsen PT, Goepfert PA, et al. A HIV-1 Gp41 peptide-liposome vaccine elicits neutralizing epitope-targeted antibody responses in healthy individuals. medRxiv. 2024

Chapter 3

Perspective Chapter: The Role of Basophils and Eosinophils in Arbovirus Infection Diseases

Valeria Vargas, Mariana Segovia-Mendoza and Jorge Cime-Castillo

Abstract

Arbovirus infections, including those caused by flavivirus, such as dengue and Zika viruses, as well as alphaviruses like chikungunya, continue to pose significant global health challenges. Within the context of arboviral infectious diseases, innate immune cells, including mast cells, basophils, and eosinophils, play a pivotal role in the pathogenesis of these viral infections. This chapter aims to elucidate the roles of eosinophils, basophils, and mast cells as mediators between innate and adaptive immunity, highlighting their involvement in tissue damage mechanisms during infection and their contribution to stimulating both humoral and cellular immune responses. In certain instances, these cells may act as reservoirs, facilitating viral replication and dissemination within the host. A comprehensive understanding of these mechanisms holds potential for advancing therapeutic, diagnostic, and prognostic strategies.

Keywords: arbovirus infection disease, cellular innate immune, pathogenesis, viral replication, potential diagnostic strategies

1. Introduction

The innate immune system functions as the primary barrier to external threats and pathogens, mounting a rapid, cell-mediated response through effector cells such as NK cells, mast cells, neutrophils, basophils, eosinophils, dendritic cells, monocytes, and macrophages. Beyond direct pathogen clearance, these cells play a pivotal role in activating and shaping the adaptive immune response. Signaling plays a crucial role in determining which immunological modules are activated, thereby customizing the immune response to target specific groups of pathogens that invade the host. The innate immune system is composed of myeloid cells and lymphoid cells (ILCs). Like T and B cells, ILCs, which include natural killer (NK) cells, originate from common lymphoid progenitor cells [1]. Myeloid cells comprise macrophages, dendritic cells, monocytes, and granulocytes, including eosinophils, basophils, and neutrophils. While neutrophils and macrophages have been linked to microbial infections, other granulocytes and mast cells have been mostly associated with helminth infections;

IntechOpen

however, it is now known that these cell types are often activated in response to a wide range of microbial and multicellular pathogens [1]. Basophils are granulocytes derived from bone marrow precursor cells and released into the blood circulation. It is known that basophils are the major effector cells of type I hypersensitivity responses responsible for anaphylaxis, asthma, and other allergic disorders. These cells share numerous standard functions with mast cells, including the elaboration of preformed and newly synthesized mediators, as well as the expression of cytokines that drive Th2 inflammation, such as IL-4. They also possess Toll-like receptors, complement receptors, and numerous other cytokine and chemokine receptors that endow them with an expanded role in the innate and adaptive immune components of allergic inflammation. Eosinophils, on the other hand, accumulate in mucoid tissue in processes induced by allergenic inflammation by the activation of adhesion molecules like VCAM-1 and VLA-4. The most important factor for the growth, differentiation, and specific release of eosinophils from the bone marrow is IL-5. Activated eosinophils are equipped with uniquely toxic molecules that are synthesized and stored in intracellular granules, such as major basic protein (MBP), which has antihelminthic activity. Other important eosinophil-derived molecules include peroxides that generate local tissue damage, as well as pro-inflammatory leukotrienes, prostaglandins, and platelet-activating factor (**Figure 1**).

As mentioned above, in the first instance, eosinophils and basophils were considered immune response cells specialized in defense against parasites; however, it is now

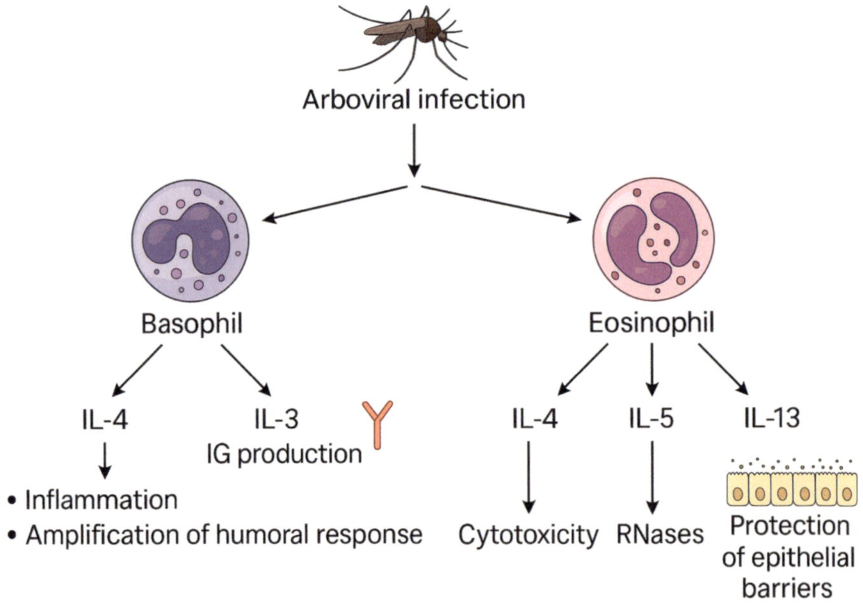

Figure 1.
Arboviral infection: Immunological mechanisms involving basophils and eosinophils during arboviral infections are critical to understanding the host response to pathogens such as dengue, Zika, and chikungunya viruses. Basophils play a significant role in enhancing the humoral immune responses by facilitating immunoglobulin production through IL-3 induction and promoting Th2 inflammation via IL-4 mediation. Concurrently, eosinophils exhibit antiviral properties through IL-4-driven cytotoxicity, IL-5-mediated ribonuclease release, and IL-13-associated enhancement of epithelial barrier integrity. These processes underscore the dual function of granulocytes in modulating both protective and pathological immune responses in the context of arboviral diseases.

known that both are also involved in an antiviral response. For instance, eosinophils are recruited to the lungs in response to the respiratory syncytial virus. These eosinophils express Toll-like receptors (TLRs) that recognize viral nucleic acids, leading to their activation and degranulation following the recognition of single-stranded RNA via TLR7-MyD88 [2]. Similarly, the involvement of eosinophils in the attenuation of parainfluenza 1 virus through the production of nitric oxide has been documented [3]. The activation of eosinophils can mitigate inflammation induced by SARS-CoV-2, releasing cytokines such as IL-13 and antiviral granular proteins, including eosinophil-derived neurotoxins and eosinophil cationic protein, in addition to functioning as antigen-presenting cells. On the other hand, eosinophil accumulation in the lungs may cause tissue injury driven by leptin and gamma interferon (IFN-γ).

Moreover, eosinophils can regulate adaptive immunity by engaging T cells through membrane-bound interactions and by producing soluble mediators that modulate T-cell responses. Notably, a low eosinophil count (eosinopenia) has been reported in patients hospitalized with COVID-19 [4]. The decline in eosinophil levels is more frequently observed in patients with the alpha and omicron variants, with levels lower than those in patients infected with other unrelated viruses [5]. This eosinopenia may result from decreased eosinophil production or suppression of their functionality related to movement and activity. However, there is also the possibility that SARS-CoV-2 infects eosinophils via CD147, an immunomodulatory receptor associated as a co-receptor of SARS-CoV-2 [6]. In SARS-CoV-2-infected patients, eosinophils display high levels of CD147; however, activated eosinophils in critically ill individuals exhibit diminished CD147 expression, possibly as a result of viral adsorption [7]. Metapneumoviruses can also be modulated by neurotoxins and cationic proteins, which also exhibit RNAse activity as derivatives of activated eosinophils [8].

Conversely, basophils, traditionally regarded as minor contributors to the immune response, demonstrate significant involvement in HIV infection. When activated, they prompt the release of viral antigens, cytokines, and immune complexes, which subsequently influence cytokine release and the activation of adaptive immune cells. Moreover, basophils serve as antigen-presenting cells, which affects the spread of the virus and contributes to immune dysregulation. Basophils play a crucial role in controlling HIV infection by releasing cytokines, particularly IL-3, IL-4, and IL-13, which are involved in the differentiation, antibody production, and polarization of immune cells. Similarly, a direct correlation has been observed between basophils and disease progression in patients positive for SARS-CoV-2, where the induction of IL-13 production aids in reducing inflammation and promoting an antibody-dependent response to the virus [9]. Additionally, the influenza A virus induces the release of histamine from basophils through the activity of the virus's neuraminidase [10].

While the involvement of eosinophils and basophils in the immune response to various viruses is well-established, their specific contributions to the defense against arboviruses remain largely unexplored.

The arboviral infections (viruses transmitted by arthropods such as mosquitoes) represent an emerging public health problem in tropical and subtropical regions. Among the most relevant arboviruses are dengue (DENV), Zika (ZIKV), and chikungunya (CHIKV), which share transmission mechanisms and part of their pathogenesis, but differ in their immunological and clinical consequences. Although most studies have focused on lymphocytes, monocytes/macrophages, and dendritic cells, the contribution of granulocytes such as eosinophils and basophils has begun to gain interest, especially due to their potential modulatory role in innate immunity, in the transition to adaptive responses, and immunopathological phenomena [11].

Therefore, this chapter examines the roles of eosinophils and basophils in arboviral infections, with a particular emphasis on their immunomodulatory and pro-inflammatory functions.

1.1 Dengue virus infection

Dengue fever is an arboviral disease transmitted by mosquitoes, resulting from infection with the dengue virus. The virus utilizes its structural protein (E) to identify and bind to its receptors, which include a variety of high- and low-affinity receptors such as DC-SIGN, mannose receptor, GRP78, heparan sulfate, and Fcγ receptors, particularly implicated in secondary infections. These receptors function as binding proteins, facilitating viral entry into host cells. However, it is posited that multiple receptors may be involved in mediating the entry of DENV into a single cell [12]. This process initiates several cellular reactions and activates the immune system.

Upon infecting the host cell, the virus releases the membrane protein (M) and targets Langerhans cells. Once the dendritic cells are infected, the virus begins to spread to various types of blood cells. This includes different white blood cells such as lymphocytes, basophils, eosinophils, neutrophils, monocytes, and macrophages, as well as platelets and erythrocytes. Subsequently, the virus targets monocytes or macrophages for replication, eventually invading vascular endothelial cells (endotheliocytes), liver cells (hepatocytes), tissue macrophages (Kupffer cells), and bone marrow stromatic cells. This invasion enhances endothelial permeability, potentially leading to the overproduction of matrix metalloproteinases (MMP) and other cellular mediators. Once all monocyte blood cells are infected, the response to NK, IFNγ, and tumor necrosis factor alpha (TNF-α) cells is activated, with various pattern recognition receptors, such as TL3, playing a role in virus recognition and the activation of innate immunity.

Additionally, the MDA5 protein may act as a cytosolic sensor that detects double-stranded viral RNA, subsequently triggering the transcription of genes encoding type I interferon (IFN) and RIG-I (retinoic acid-inducible I gene). Furthermore, viral non-structural proteins such as NS1 interfere with the endothelial glycocalyx by upregulating three of the four cytosolic (Neu 2), plasma membrane (Neu 3), and lysosomal (Neu 1) endothelial sialidases. These sialidases translocate to the plasma membrane, leading to the hydrolysis of the endothelial glycocalyx layer that expresses sialic acid residues, thereby disrupting the endothelial layer and ultimately exacerbating the pathogenesis of dengue fever. Collectively, the various molecules of the dengue virus activate different cellular components of the immune cells, resulting in immune dysfunctions and contributing to the severe pathogenesis of dengue.

1.2 Zika virus infection

The Zika virus (ZIKV), similar to the DENV virus, is a member of the Flaviviridae family and is characterized as a positive-sense RNA virus with an approximate genome size of 11 kb. This virus shows a particular affinity for infecting neural progenitor cells [13], and it has been implicated in the development of microcephaly and other neural developmental disorders. Additionally, ZIKV has been associated with Guillain-Barré syndrome, a condition marked by ascending paralysis and polyneuropathy [14]. The virus exhibits tropism for various cell types, including endothelial cells in the placenta and vaginal epithelium, neural progenitors, astrocytes, optic nerve cells, Sertoli cells in the testicles, and peripheral dendritic cells. Research has demonstrated that ZIKV can replicate in macrophages, trophoblasts, and endothelial cells of the placenta, although monocytes have been identified as the initial target of ZIKV in peripheral blood [15]. Studies involving both human and animal models have shown that ZIKV infection can lead to the persistence of the virus and its genetic material in various body fluids, such as semen, saliva, tears, and urine, as well as in target organs, including immuno-privileged sites like the eyes, brain, and testicles, and the female genital tract [16]. In addition to receptors identified for other flaviviruses, ZIKV can recognize its target cells through receptors such as T-cell immunoglobulin and mucin domain 1 (TIM-1) and Mer receptors of the TAM family (Tyro 3, AXL) by binding to the virus's envelope protein. Receptors such as CCR7 and RAGE have been implicated in the migration of infected monocytes across the blood-brain barrier, facilitating infection of central nervous system tissue [17]. Upon entry into the central nervous system, monocytes can transmit the virus to resident neural cells, thereby contributing to neuropathogenesis.

After the receptor is identified, the virus penetrates the cell through clathrin-mediated endocytosis, similar to the mechanism used by other flaviviruses, to release its genome into the cytoplasm. Viral replication then takes place on the endoplasmic reticulum (ER) surface. Studies using electron microscopy have shown that Zika virus replication is restricted to ER compartments within astroglial cells and neurons, suggesting a membrane-associated replication process [18]. Once inside the cell, ZIKV is detected by intracellular receptors like Toll-like receptors and RIG-I-like receptors, which recognize viral RNA and trigger a signaling cascade. This cascade activates transcription factors, interferon regulatory factors, and mitogen-activated protein kinases, which boost the production of pro-inflammatory and antiviral molecules, including cytokines (IL-6, IL-8, IL-1β, and TNF-α), chemokines (CCL2 and CXCL10), and antiviral proteins (IFIT1 and RSAD2/viperin) [19]. These molecules work to suppress viral replication, provoke inflammation, and attract immune cells to the infection site). During the acute phase of infection, the virus stimulates the expression of inflammatory genes like TNFα, IL-6, and IL-1β. Among the immune effectors, CD8 cytotoxic T lymphocytes are crucial in eradicating ZIKV-infected cells and coordinating an antiviral immune response by secreting IFNγ and TNFα, thereby enhancing the immune response by activating antigen-presenting macrophages and promoting GM-CSF [20].

2. Eosinophils in arboviral infections

2.1 General biology

Eosinophils are a type of granular white blood cell that originates in the bone marrow, influenced by IL-5, IL-3, and GM-CSF (granulocyte-macrophage colony-stimulating factor). After circulating briefly in the bloodstream, they move to peripheral tissues [21]. Traditionally known for defending against helminths, eosinophils also play roles in antiviral defense, inflammation regulation, and tissue remodeling. Their granules contain cytotoxic proteins like eosinophil cationic protein (ECP), major basic protein (MBP), and eosinophil peroxidase (EPO), which have direct antiviral and cytolytic effects [22]. Additionally, eosinophils release a wide array of cytokines and chemokines and can form extracellular traps (EETs), aiding in pathogen containment and immune regulation [23]. These cells are equipped with various membrane molecules and cellular mediators that enable them to function effectively in their environment. Express numerous receptors for pathogen-associated molecular patterns (PAMPs) and damage-associated molecular patterns (DAMPs), cytokines, chemokines, proteases, immunoglobulins, and lipid mediators, facilitating their migration, survival, and interaction with other immune cells. These interactions are mediated by adhesion molecules, notably surface integrins and selectins. When activated, eosinophils degranulate, releasing granule contents such as major basic protein (MBP), eosinophil peroxidase (EPO), eosinophil-derived neurotoxin (EDN), along with lipid mediators, cytokines, and chemokines. These mediators play essential roles in thrombotic environments and inflammatory conditions. Their activity is tightly regulated by inhibitory receptors that limit eosinophil function [7].

2.2 Eosinophils in dengue (DENV)

Marked eosinopenia has been documented during the acute phase of dengue, possibly due to tissue migration, apoptosis induced by pro-inflammatory cytokines (IFN-γ and TNF-α), or transient bone marrow suppression [24]. Recovery of eosinophil counts predicts favorable resolution, while persistent eosinopenia could correlate with vascular extravasation and shock [25, 26]. Eosinophils can release RNases and act as antigen-presenting cells ([27]; **Table 1**).

2.2.1 Clinical observations

Studies in patients with acute dengue have documented significant eosinopenia during the early febrile phase, with progressive recovery in the convalescent phase. This eosinopenia has been correlated with clinical severity, including cases of severe dengue and plasma leak syndrome. Eosinopenia has been observed in the acute phase of the disease, and a rebound increase in eosinophils has been noted with an increase in the absolute eosinophil count [28].

2.2.2 Potential mechanisms

Tissue migration: it has been suggested that eosinophils migrate from the circulation to inflamed tissues, such as the lung and gastrointestinal tract. i) Viral cytokine-induced apoptosis: elevated levels of TNF-α and IFN-γ can induce eosinophilic apoptosis. ii) Immunomodulatory effect: there is evidence that eosinophils contribute to the modulation of the Th1/Th2 response, affecting the immunopathology of dengue.

2.2.3 Clinical implications

Eosinophil count can be an indirect marker of clinical progression. Its recovery has been proposed as an indicator of favorable disease resolution [29–31].

2.3 Eosinophils in Zika (ZIKV)

ZIKV infection has been linked to neurological issues, such as Guillain-Barré syndrome, and congenital abnormalities in newborns [32]. While the exact role of eosinophils in ZIKV infection is not completely understood, there is indirect evidence pointing to their participation in immunomodulatory activities.

Characteristics	Dengue (DENV)	Zika (ZIKV)	Chikungunya (CHIKV)
Peripheral cell count	Marked eosinopenia in the acute febrile phase; recovery in convalescence	Normal or mild eosinophilia in late phases; eosinopenia infrequent	Normal cell count in the acute phase; mild–moderate eosinophilia in the subacute/chronic phase
Mechanism of alteration	Tissue migration by eotaxins; TNF-α/IFN-γ-mediated apoptosis; transient bone marrow suppression	Mucosal redistribution; possible chemotaxis by IL-33 and alarmins in skin and mucosal tissues	Shift to inflamed synovium; shift to late Th2 profile
Cytokine profile	↓ Th1 (IL-2, IFN-γ) in eosinopenia; ↑ IL-10/TGF-β in critical phases	↑ IL-4 and IL-13 in neuro and placental tissues; modest IFN-α production	↑ IL-5/IL-13 in chronic phase; coexistence with IL-17/TNF-α in persistent arthritis
Effector functions	Release of ECP, MBP, and EPO with antiviral activity; antigen presentation (MHC II)	Protection of epithelial barriers (CNS, placenta); secretion of antiviral RNases	Moderate cytotoxicity in synovial fluid; dual participation in inflammation and tissue repair
Clinical implications	Prognostic marker: eosinophil recovery anticipates resolution phase; persistence is associated with risk of extravasation.	Not commendable as a standard biomarker; possible correlate with cutaneous manifestations and neuroprotection	Potential indicator of chronic arthritis; Candidate for monitoring response to modulatory therapies
Potential therapeutic targets	IL-5 modulators or eotaxin receptor antagonists.	Strategies to enhance antiviral RNases at immune barriers.	Anti-IL-5 (e.g., mepolizumab) or blockade of eotaxins in late stages to control inflammation.

Table 1.
Comparison of eosinophil participation in arbovirus infections.

Studies using mouse models with induced eosinophilia have demonstrated improved antiviral responses against respiratory syncytial virus (RSV) infection. However, their contribution to enhancing antiviral host defense is still uncertain, as indicated by reduced viral loads and tissue damage, which suggests a possible protective function; nonetheless, their role in bolstering antiviral host defense remains ambiguous. While direct studies on ZIKV are lacking, increased serum IL-5 and eotaxin levels in patients with severe disease manifestations suggest eosinophil mobilization. Eosinophil interactions with ZIKV-infected epithelial or endothelial cells could modulate local inflammatory responses, potentially influencing viral dissemination and disease severity, especially in the central nervous system and the placenta ([33, 34]; **Table 1**).

2.3.1 Preliminary findings

Unlike dengue, eosinopenia in Zika has not been systematically reported. Limited studies suggest that the role of eosinophils may be less prominent in acute ZIKV infection [34]. Given the association of Zika with neurological and congenital complications, further study of the interaction of eosinophils with glial and placental cells is required.

2.4 Eosinophils in chikungunya (CHIKV)

CHIKV infection typically causes intense joint inflammation, fever, and myalgia. The chronic phase may persist for months or even years, substantially impacting patients' quality of life [35–37]. In this context, eosinophils may play a dual role. In the acute phase, eosinopenia is frequently observed, likely due to eosinophil migration to inflamed tissues. Eosinophilic infiltration has been documented in skin and synovial biopsies, supporting their involvement in local inflammation [38].

Eosinophils may contribute both to viral clearance and chronic inflammation by releasing cytotoxic granules that damage tissues and perpetuate the inflammatory process. Furthermore, their ability to secrete pro-inflammatory mediators and present antigens may amplify T- and B-cell activation within inflamed joints ([39]; **Table 1**).

2.4.1 Reactive eosinophilia

In contrast to dengue and Zika, some studies have reported mild eosinophilia in the subacute or chronic phases of chikungunya infection, associated with persistent joint inflammation [39]. In post-acute phases, a shift in the immune profile may occur that favors eosinophil expansion. Eosinophils may contribute to chronic pathology by releasing pro-inflammatory enzymes and cytokines in the inflamed synovium.

2.4.2 Therapeutic implications

Chikungunya virus (CHIKV) is part of a widespread group of alphaviruses known for causing long-lasting polyarthritis or arthralgia, which current treatments often fail to adequately address. These arthritic symptoms are commonly linked to increased levels of the chemokine CCL2 [Chemokine (C-C motif)] and a significant infiltration of monocytes/macrophages. There are several inhibitors in development that target CCL2 and its receptor CCR2 (Chemokine (C-C motif) receptor 2), which could potentially be used to treat certain inflammatory conditions, including autoimmune and viral arthritis. Poo et al. [2014, 39] conducted a study using CCR2/mice to explore the effects of CCR2 deficiency on CHIKV infection. In these CCR2/mice, the usual monocyte/macrophage infiltration was replaced by a marked presence of neutrophils, followed by eosinophils, along with changes in the expression of various inflammatory mediators such as IL-1, IL-10, granulocyte colony-stimulating factor, CXCL1, and CXCL2. Although the recruitment of CCR2 and monocytes can intensify inflammation, it also seems crucial for reducing severe pathology and resolving inflammation after an alphavirus infection.

3. Basophils in arboviral infections

3.1 General biology

Comprising less than 1% of the leukocytes in the bloodstream, basophils are identified by their cytoplasmic granules, which contain histamine used in managing alphaviral arthritides. They secrete IL-4 and IL-13, participating in humoral immunity and allergic responses, and express high-affinity receptors for IgE (FcεRI), linking them to allergic reactions. Still, they are also involved in immune modulation during parasitic and viral infections [40].

A key feature of basophils is their capacity to release soluble mediators such as IL-4, IL-13, histamine, and leukotrienes, which positions them as both effector and regulatory cells. Furthermore, their ability to induce T helper 2 (Th2) polarization of $CD4^+$ T cells has been documented, which may influence the course of viral infections ([41]; **Figure 2**).

3.2 Basophil activation during DENV infection

Recent studies have demonstrated basophil activation during acute DENV infection, particularly around the critical phase (days 4–6 post-symptom onset), coinciding with plasma leakage and endothelial dysfunction (**Figure 2**). Potential mechanisms for activation include i) immune complex-mediated stimulation: In secondary infections, subneutralizing antibodies may form immune complexes with DENV, leading to basophil activation via FcγRII; ii) cytokine-driven expansion and priming: IL-3, GM-CSF, and thymic stromal lymphopoietin (TSLP) promote basophil proliferation and functional activation; iii) paracrine signals from infected cells: Basophils may be indirectly activated by cytokines and alarmins released by DENV-infected monocytes or dendritic cells ([42, 43]; **Table 2**).

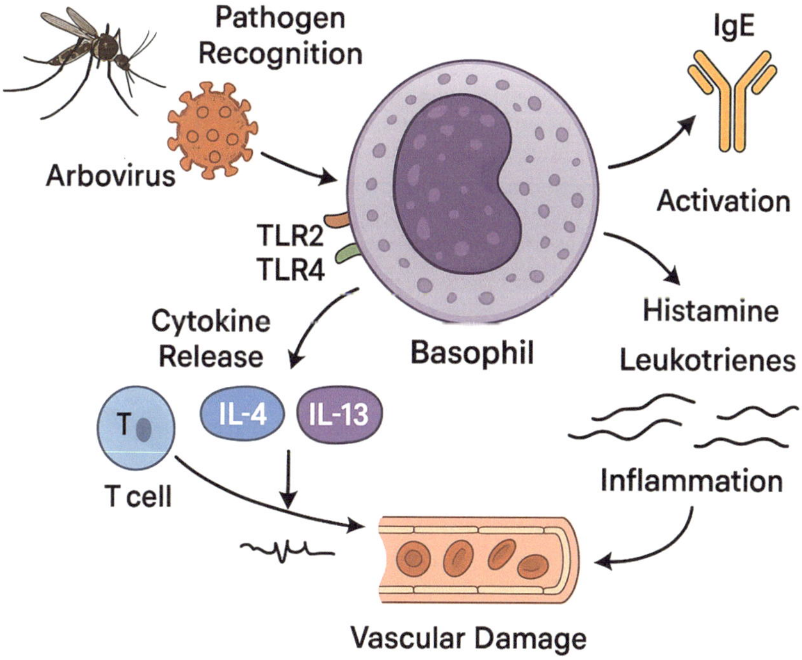

Figure 2.
Basophil activation in arboviral infections: Immunological mechanisms involving basophils in arboviral infections. Upon recognition of arboviral components via Toll-like receptors (TLR2/TLR4), basophils become activated and release pro-inflammatory mediators, including interleukin-4 (IL-4), interleukin-13 (IL-13), histamine, and leukotrienes. These mediators contribute to vascular permeability, tissue inflammation, and recruitment of T lymphocytes. Additionally, IgE-mediated activation through FceRI may amplify basophil responses, exacerbating the immunopathogenesis observed in severe arboviral disease.

Characteristics	Dengue (DENV)	Zika (ZIKV)	Chikungunya (CHIKV)
Basophil activation	During the critical phase (4–6 days post-infection)	During acute phase and in neurological cases	Possible; limited evidence
Main activation mechanism	Immune complexes (FcγR), IL-3, signals from infected cells	Proinflammatory cytokines, IL-33, TSLP	Indirect PRRs, IL-3-mediated activation
Cytokines produced	IL-4, IL-13, CCL3, CCL4	IL-4, IL-13 (associated with BBB* disruption)	IL-4 and IL-6 (possibly linked to pain and arthralgia)
Vasoactive mediators	Histamine, leukotrienes → vascular leakage	Histamine → BBB dysfunction, rash	Histamine, prostaglandins → edema, synovitis
Primary immunological role	Promotes Th2 polarization; enhances vascular permeability	Neuroinflammatory modulator; alters immune polarization	Possible amplifier of synovial inflammation
Clinical or experimental evidence	Elevated CD63, CD203c, IL-4, tryptase in DH/DSS	Basophil activation in peripheral blood; elevated CNS histamine	Some evidence in murine models; limited in humans

**BBB: Blood-brain barrier.*

Table 2.
Comparison of basophil participation in arbovirus infections.

3.2.1 Immunomodulatory functions of basophils in DENV

Basophils contribute to dengue pathogenesis via multiple mechanisms: i) Vascular permeability enhancement: Basophil-derived histamine and leukotrienes C4/D4 increase endothelial permeability, a hallmark of severe dengue. Elevated serum histamine levels correlate with disease severity and the onset of vascular leakage in DSS patients [44]. ii) Promotion of Th2 skewing: IL-4 and IL-13 released by basophils promote Th2 polarization, which may suppress antiviral Th1 responses, diminish cytotoxic CD8+ T-cell activity, and impair IFN-γ-mediated viral clearance [45]. iii) Crosstalk with antigen-presenting cells: Human basophils can influence dendritic cell maturation and antigen presentation, thereby modulating the initiation and polarization of adaptive immune responses ([46, 47]; **Figure 2**).

3.2.2 Clinical evidence

Kwissa et al. [48] demonstrated that basophils migrate to infection sites in murine models and amplify IL-4 production in draining lymph nodes. In human studies, basophils exhibit increased surface expression of CD63 and CD203c during the critical phase of dengue infection. These findings correlate with elevated plasma IL-4 levels and disease severity. Additionally, increased serum histamine and tryptase—markers of degranulation shared by mast cells and basophils—have been reported in DHF patients, suggesting coordinated activation of granule-containing effector cells.

3.2.3 Therapeutic and diagnostic implications

IL-4/IL-13 blockade: Monoclonal antibodies such as dupilumab may reduce Th2-mediated inflammation [49]. Basophil membrane stabilizers: Agents like sodium cromoglycate or ketotifen could prevent basophil degranulation and mediator release [44, 50]. Monitoring activated basophils using flow cytometry or quantifying serum IL-4/IL-13 levels may provide early prognostic indicators of disease progression in DENV-infected individuals [29, 51, 52].

3.3 Basophil activation during Zika infection

Zika virus (ZIKV), an arbovirus belonging to the Flavivirus genus, has emerged as a major public health concern in recent decades. Although its clinical presentation is often mild, ZIKV infection has been associated with severe complications such as Guillain-Barré syndrome and congenital malformations, including microcephaly. The immune response to ZIKV has been extensively investigated, particularly the roles of T lymphocytes, monocytes, macrophages, and dendritic cells. However, the contribution of less abundant innate immune cells such as basophils has only recently gained attention due to their regulatory functions in viral infections, hypersensitivity reactions, and modulation of adaptive immunity (**Table 2**).

3.3.1 Evidence of basophil involvement in ZIKV infections

Although direct studies on basophil-ZIKV interactions are limited, emerging evidence suggests that these leukocytes may participate in the course of infection through both direct and indirect mechanisms: i) Activation by Viral Components, basophils can be activated in the presence of viral particles or viral proteins, including those derived from ZIKV [53]. Such activation may lead to the release of pro-inflammatory cytokines such as IL-4 and TNF-α, thereby amplifying inflammation and promoting the recruitment of other immune cells. ii) Production of IL-4 and IL-13, in ZIKV infection, this could play a dual role, promoting resolution of inflammation on one hand, while negatively modulating antiviral Th1 and NK cell responses on the other [54, 55]. iii) Tissue Infiltration and Role in Immunopathology, animal studies have shown that basophils can infiltrate affected tissues during viral infections. Although direct evidence in ZIKV remains scarce, basophilic infiltration in tissues such as the skin, placenta, or nervous system may contribute to immunopathological processes, including barrier disruption and pro-inflammatory cell recruitment ([56]; **Figure 2**).

3.3.2 Clinical and therapeutic implications

The potential involvement of basophils in ZIKV infection opens new avenues for diagnostic and therapeutic approaches. Monitoring basophil activation using assays such as the Basophil Activation Test (BAT) may provide early biomarkers of inflammation or disease prognosis. Furthermore, pharmacological modulation of basophil function—using histamine receptor antagonists, IL-4 inhibitors, or monoclonal anti-IgE antibodies—could be evaluated as adjunctive strategies to reduce inflammatory or neurological complications [57].

3.4 Basophils in chikungunya (CHIKV)

Chikungunya virus (CHIKV), an arbovirus belonging to the Alphavirus genus (family Togaviridae), has emerged as a significant global public health threat due to its capacity to cause explosive outbreaks and debilitating clinical syndromes, including fever, persistent arthralgia, and inflammatory manifestations. While our understanding of CHIKV immunopathogenesis has advanced, the involvement of innate effector cells such as basophils has received limited attention. Nevertheless, emerging evidence suggests that basophils may play a substantial role in the development and persistence of inflammation during CHIKV infection ([58]; **Table 2**).

3.4.1 Possible mechanisms of basophil activation in CHIKV infection

Although CHIKV does not directly infect basophils, these cells can become activated in the inflammatory microenvironment generated during infection:
i) Pro-inflammatory cytokine signaling: in the acute phase of CHIKV infection, elevated levels of IL-1β, IL-6, TNF-α, and IL-3 may promote basophil activation and expansion [59, 60]. ii) Activation of IL-33 and TSLP: epithelial-derived alarmins, released from damaged synovial or cutaneous tissues, can rapidly activate basophils, promoting Th2-type inflammation [60–62]. iii) Immune complex engagement: in secondary infections, the presence of virus-specific IgG or IgE antibodies may lead to the formation of immune complexes that activate basophils via FcγR or FcεRI ([63–65]; **Figure 2**).

4. Conclusion

Eosinophils and basophils are integral to the pathophysiology of arboviral infections, contributing not only to tissue damage and immunopathology but also to defense mechanisms, tissue repair, and immune regulation. A deeper understanding of their behavior could facilitate the development of more precise diagnostic and therapeutic strategies. Although eosinophils have not traditionally been considered central to the pathogenesis of viral infections such as dengue, Zika, or chikungunya, their regulatory function within the immune response is gaining recognition. A comprehensive understanding of their roles throughout the various stages of these diseases could inform novel strategies for clinical management and aid in the development of more targeted therapeutic interventions. Historically overlooked in the context of viral infections, basophils are now acknowledged as significant modulators of dengue pathogenesis. They emerge as potential targets for therapeutic intervention and as biomarkers for severe disease outcomes due to their capacity to influence adaptive immunity, promote systemic inflammation, and disrupt vascular integrity. Continued research into their precise roles may yield novel insights into the immunopathophysiology of dengue and inform the development of targeted therapeutic strategies. Basophils, long neglected in the context of viral infections, are emerging as key modulators of immune responses in ZIKV infection. Their ability to secrete cytokines, interact with antigen-specific IgE, and shape both innate and adaptive immunity positions them as potential contributors to antiviral defense and pathogenesis. Further studies are warranted to elucidate their precise roles in ZIKV infection and explore their utility in diagnostic and therapeutic strategies. Although underexplored, basophils are increasingly recognized as key immunomodulatory players in CHIKV pathogenesis, particularly during the inflammatory and chronic phases of the disease. Their ability to influence immune polarization, promote persistent inflammation, and shape the tissue microenvironment underscores their relevance in host defense and immunopathology.

Acknowledgements

We express our gratitude to the Department of Pharmacology at the Faculty of Medicine, National Autonomous University of Mexico, and the Center for Research on Infectious Diseases at the National Institute of Public Health for their support.

Conflict of interest

The authors declare no conflict of interest.

Author details

Valeria Vargas[1], Mariana Segovia-Mendoza[1] and Jorge Cime-Castillo[2]*

1 Laboratory of Endocrine Pharmacology, Department of Pharmacology, Faculty of Medicine, National Autonomous University of Mexico, Mexico City, Mexico

2 Center for Research on Infectious Diseases, National Institute of Public Health, Cuernavaca, Mexico

*Address all correspondence to: jorge.cime@insp.mx

References

[1] Rivera A, Siracusa MC, Yap GS, Gause WC. Innate cell communication kick-starts pathogen-specific immunity. Nature Immunology. 2016;**17**(4):356-363. DOI: 10.1038/ni.3375

[2] Phipps S, Lam CE, Mahalingam S, Newhouse M, Ramirez R, Rosenberg HF, et al. Eosinophils contribute to innate antiviral immunity and promote clearance of respiratory syncytial virus. Blood. 2007;**110**(5):1578-1586. DOI: 10.1182/blood-2007-01-071340

[3] Drake MG, Bivins-Smith ER, Proskocil BJ, Nie Z, Scott GD, Lee JJ, et al. Human and mouse eosinophils have antiviral activity against parainfluenza virus. American Journal of Respiratory Cell and Molecular Biology. 2016;**55**(3):387-394. DOI: 10.1165/rcmb.2015-0405OC

[4] Zhang JJ, Dong X, Cao YY, Yuan YD, Yang YB, Yan YQ, et al. Clinical characteristics of 140 patients infected with SARS-CoV-2 in Wuhan, China. Allergy. 2020;**75**(7):1730-1741. DOI: 10.1111/all.14238

[5] Zhu Z, Cai J, Tang Q, Mo YY, Deng T, Zhang X, et al. Circulating eosinophils associated with responsiveness to COVID-19 vaccine and the disease severity in patients with SARS-CoV-2 omicron variant infection. BMC Pulmonary Medicine. 2023;**23**(1):177. DOI: 10.1186/s12890-023-02473-w

[6] Wang Y, Wang Y, Luo W, Huang L, Xiao J, Li F, et al. A comprehensive investigation of the mRNA and protein level of ACE2, the putative receptor of SARS-CoV-2, in human tissues and blood cells. International Journal of Medical Sciences. 2020;**17**(11):1522-1531. DOI: 10.7150/ijms.46695

[7] Sahli W, Vitte J, Desnues B. Eosinophils and COVID-19: Insights into immune complexity and vaccine safety. Clinical and Translational Allergy. 2025;**15**(3):e70050. DOI: 10.1002/clt2.70050

[8] Andrade CA, Pacheco GA, Gálvez NMS, Soto JA, Bueno SM, Kalergis AM. Innate immune components that regulate the pathogenesis and resolution of hRSV and hMPV infections. Viruses. 2020;**12**(6):637. DOI: 10.3390/v12060637

[9] Bonam SR, Chauvin C, Levillayer L, Mathew MJ, Sakuntabhai A, Bayry J. SARS-CoV-2 induces cytokine responses in human basophils. Frontiers in Immunology. 2022;**13**:838448. DOI: 10.3389/fimmu.2022.838448

[10] Gammeri L, Sanfilippo S, Alessandrello C, Gangemi S, Minciullo PL. Mast cells and basophils in major viral diseases: What are the correlations with SARS-CoV-2, influenza a viruses, HIV, and dengue? Cells. 2024;**13**(24):2044. DOI: 10.3390/cells13242044

[11] Rothenberg ME, Hogan SP. The eosinophil. Annual Review of Immunology. 2006;**24**:147-174. DOI: 10.1146/annurev.immunol.24.021605.090720

[12] Begum F, Das S, Mukherjee D, Mal S, Ray U. Insight into the tropism of dengue virus in humans. Viruses. 2019;**11**(12):1136. DOI: 10.3390/v11121136

[13] Tang H, Hammack C, Ogden SC, Wen Z, Qian X, Li Y, et al. Zika virus infects human cortical neural progenitors and attenuates their growth. Cell Stem

Cell. 2016;**18**(5):587-590. DOI: 10.1016/j.stem.2016.02.016

[14] Beattie J, Parajuli S, Sanger M, Lee G, Pleninger P, Crowley G, et al. Zika virus-associated Guillain-Barré syndrome in a returning US Traveler. Infectious Diseases in Clinical Practice (Baltimore, Md.). 2018;**26**(6):e80-e84. DOI: 10.1097/IPC.0000000000000654

[15] Foo SS, Chen W, Chan Y, Bowman JW, Chang LC, Choi Y, et al. Asian Zika virus strains target CD14+ blood monocytes and induce M2-skewed immunosuppression during pregnancy. Nature Microbiology. 2017;**2**(11):1558-1570. DOI: 10.1038/s41564-017-0016-3

[16] Miner JJ, Diamond MS. Zika virus pathogenesis and tissue tropism. Cell Host & Microbe. 2017;**21**(2):134-142. DOI: 10.1016/j.chom.2017.01.004

[17] Li F, Wang Y, Yu L, Cao S, Wang K, Yuan J, et al. Viral infection of the central nervous system and neuroinflammation precede blood-brain barrier disruption during Japanese encephalitis virus infection. Journal of Virology. 2015;**89**(10):5602-5614. DOI: 10.1128/JVI.00143-15

[18] Roozitalab A, Zhang J, Zhang C, Tang Q, Zhao RY. The evolving role of Zika virus envelope protein in viral entry and pathogenesis. Viruses. 2025;**17**(6):817. DOI: 10.3390/v17060817

[19] Santana LMB, de Moura IA, Mouzinho Ramos Tanaka Y, França RFO. Zika virus: A review of biology, clinical impacts, and coinfections. Viruses. 2025;**17**(5):637. DOI: 10.3390/v17050637

[20] Park S. CD8 T cell dynamics and immune cell trafficking in ZIKV infection: Implications for neuroinflammation and therapy. Virology Journal. 2025;**22**(1):242. DOI: 10.1186/s12985-025-02866-9

[21] Rosenberg HF, Dyer KD, Foster PS. Eosinophils: Changing perspectives in health and disease. Nature Reviews Immunology. 2013;**13**(1):9-22. DOI: 10.1038/nri3341

[22] Jacobsen EA, Taranova AG, Lee NA, Lee JJ. Eosinophils: Singularly destructive effector cells or purveyors of immunoregulation? The Journal of Allergy and Clinical Immunology. 2007;**119**(6):1313-1320. DOI: 10.1016/j.jaci.2007.03.043

[23] Gazzinelli-Guimaraes PH, Dulek B, Swanson P, Lack J, Roederer M, Nutman TB. Single-cell molecular signature of pathogenic T helper subsets in type 2-associated disorders in humans. JCI Insight. 2024;**9**(7):e177720. DOI: 10.1172/jci.insight.177720

[24] Jameel T, Mehmood K, Mujtaba G, Choudhry N, Afzal N, Paul RF. Changing haematological parameters in dengue viral infections. Journal of Ayub Medical College, Abbottabad: JAMC. 2012;**24**(1):3-6

[25] Nayar S, Sriranjani B, Shanmugam P. Haematological predictors of recovery in dengue cases. National Journal of Laboratory Medicine. 2019;**8**(4):22-24. DOI: 10.7860/NJLM/2019/42082:2370

[26] Ye G, Xu Z, Yang M, Wang J, Liang J, Yin J, et al. Clinical features and transmission risk analysis of dengue virus infections in Shenzhen, during 2014-2019. Computational and Structural Biotechnology Journal. 2023;**21**:3728-3735. DOI: 10.1016/j.csbj.2023.07.001

[27] Rosenberg HF. Eosinophil-derived neurotoxin (EDN/RNase 2) and the mouse eosinophil-associated RNases (mEars): Expanding roles in promoting host defense. International Journal of Molecular Sciences.

2015;**16**(7):15442-15455. DOI: 10.3390/ijms160715442

[28] Gazzinelli-Guimaraes PH, Jones SM, Voehringer D, Mayer-Barber KD, Samarasinghe AE. Eosinophils as modulators of host defense during parasitic, fungal, bacterial, and viral infections. Journal of Leukocyte Biology. 2024;**116**(6):1301-1323. DOI: 10.1093/jleuko/qiae173

[29] Rashmi MV, Hamsaveena. Haematological and biochemical markers as predictors of dengue infection. The Malaysian Journal of Pathology. 2015;**37**(3):247-251

[30] Anwar F, Ullah S, Aziz AUR, Rehman AU, Khan J, Tayyab M, et al. Epidemiological and hematological investigation of dengue virus infection. Microbiology and Immunology. 2022;**66**(9):426-432. DOI: 10.1111/1348-0421.13018

[31] Yunitama AAD, Puspitasari M, Jatmiko SW, Fauziyah NF. Correlation of eosinophil-basophil count and ratio with length of stay in children dengue infection. In: Developing Intelligent Technology for Humanity. Proceeding book of ISETH (International Summit on Science, Technology, and Humanity). 2024. DOI: 10.23917/iseth.5486. E-ISSN: 2615-1588

[32] Brasil P, Pereira JP Jr, Moreira ME, Ribeiro Nogueira RM, Damasceno L, Wakimoto M, et al. Zika virus infection in pregnant women in Rio de Janeiro. The New England Journal of Medicine. 2016;**375**(24):2321-2334. DOI: 10.1056/NEJMoa1602412

[33] Saad T, PennaeCosta AA, de Góes FV, de Freitas M, de Almeida JV, de Santa Ignêz LJ, et al. Neurological manifestations of congenital Zika virus infection. Child's Nervous System: ChNS: Official Journal of the International Society for Pediatric Neurosurgery. 2018;**34**(1):73-78. DOI: 10.1007/s00381-017-3634-4

[34] Salmeron ACA, Bezerra WP, de Souza RLL, Pereira LC, do Nascimento LM, Branco ACCC, et al. Immunological imbalance in microcephalic children with congenital Zika virus syndrome. Medical Microbiology and Immunology. 2022;**211**(5-6):219-235. DOI: 10.1007/s00430-022-00746-5

[35] Burt FJ, Rolph MS, Rulli NE, Mahalingam S, Heise MT. Chikungunya: a re-emerging virus. Lancet (London, England). 2012;**379**(9816):662-671. DOI: 10.1016/S0140-6736(11)60281-X

[36] Suhrbier A, Jaffar-Bandjee MC, Gasque P. Arthritogenic alphaviruses--an overview. Nature Reviews Rheumatology. 2012;**8**(7):420-429. DOI: 10.1038/nrrheum.2012.64

[37] Wikan N, Smith DR. Zika virus: History of a newly emerging arbovirus. The Lancet Infectious Diseases. 2016;**16**(7):e119-e126. DOI: 10.1016/S1473-3099(16)30010-X

[38] Miner JJ, Aw-Yeang HX, Fox JM, Taffner S, Malkova ON, Oh ST, et al. Chikungunya viral arthritis in the United States: A mimic of seronegative rheumatoid arthritis. Arthritis & Rheumatology (Hoboken, N.J.). 2015;**67**(5):1214-1220. DOI: 10.1002/art.39027

[39] Poo YS, Nakaya H, Gardner J, Larcher T, Schroder WA, Le TT, et al. CCR2 deficiency promotes exacerbated chronic erosive neutrophil-dominated chikungunya virus arthritis. Journal of Virology. 2014;**88**(12):6862-6872. DOI: 10.1128/JVI.03364-13

[40] Karasuyama H, Mukai K, Obata K, Tsujimura Y, Wada T. Nonredundant roles of basophils in immunity. Annual Review of Immunology. 2011;**29**:45-69. DOI: 10.1146/annurev-immunol-031210-101257

[41] Karasuyama H, Miyake K, Yoshikawa S, Kawano Y, Yamanishi Y. How do basophils contribute to Th2 cell differentiation and allergic responses? International Immunology. 2018;**30**(9):391-396. DOI: 10.1093/intimm/dxy026

[42] King CA, Marshall JS, Alshurafa H, Anderson R. Release of vasoactive cytokines by antibody-enhanced dengue virus infection of a human mast cell/basophil line. Journal of Virology. 2000;**74**(15):7146-7150. DOI: 10.1128/jvi.74.15.7146-7150.2000

[43] King CA, Anderson R, Marshall JS. Dengue virus selectively induces human mast cell chemokine production. Journal of Virology. 2002;**76**(16):8408-8419. DOI: 10.1128/jvi.76.16.8408-8419.2002

[44] Silva T, Jeewandara C, Gomes L, Gangani C, Mahapatuna SD, Pathmanathan T, et al. Urinary leukotrienes and histamine in patients with varying severity of acute dengue. PLoS One. 2021;**16**(2):e0245926. DOI: 10.1371/journal.pone.0245926

[45] Karasuyama H, Yamanishi Y. Basophils have emerged as a key player in immunity. Current Opinion in Immunology. 2014;**31**:1-7. DOI: 10.1016/j.coi.2014.07.004

[46] Sokol CL, Chu NQ, Yu S, Nish SA, Laufer TM, Medzhitov R. Basophils function as antigen-presenting cells for an allergen-induced T helper type 2 response. Nature Immunology. 2009;**10**(7):713-720. DOI: 10.1038/ni.1738

[47] Nakanishi K. Basophils are potent antigen-presenting cells that selectively induce Th2 cells. European Journal of Immunology. 2010;**40**(7):1836-1842. DOI: 10.1002/eji.201040588

[48] Kwissa M, Nakaya HI, Onlamoon N, Wrammert J, Villinger F, Perng GC, et al. Dengue virus infection induces expansion of a CD14(+)CD16(+) monocyte population that stimulates plasmablast differentiation. Cell Host & Microbe. 2014;**16**(1):115-127. DOI: 10.1016/j.chom.2014.06.001

[49] Le Floc'h A, Allinne J, Nagashima K, Scott G, Birchard D, Asrat S, et al. Dual blockade of IL-4 and IL-13 with dupilumab, an IL-4Rα antibody, is required to broadly inhibit type 2 inflammation. Allergy. 2020;**75**(5):1188-1204. DOI: 10.1111/all.14151

[50] Mancel E, Drouet M, Sabbah A. Les stabilisateurs de membrane (cromones et kétotifène) [Membrane stabilizers (chromones and ketotifen)]. Allergie et Immunologie. 1999;**31**(4):103-105

[51] Manuel K, Ambroise MM, Ramdas A, Varghese RG. Pseudobasophilia as a screening tool in dengue: A Single Center Study. Journal of Laboratory Physicians. 2021;**13**(2):156-161. DOI: 10.1055/s-0041-1730849

[52] Bhattarai BR, Mishra A, Aryal S, Chhusyabaga M, Bhujel R. Association of hematological and biochemical parameters with serological markers of acute dengue infection during the 2022 dengue outbreak in Nepal. Journal of Tropical Medicine. 2023;**2023**:2904422. DOI: 10.1155/2023/2904422

[53] Coish JM, Crozier RWE, Schieffelin JS, Coorssen JR, Hunter FF, MacNeil AJ. Zika virus replication in a mast cell model is augmented by dengue virus antibody-dependent enhancement

and features a selective immune mediator secretory profile. Microbiology Spectrum. 2022;**10**(4):e0177222. DOI: 10.1128/spectrum.01772-22

[54] Min B, Prout M, Hu-Li J, Zhu J, Jankovic D, Morgan ES, et al. Basophils produce IL-4 and accumulate in tissues after infection with a Th2-inducing parasite. The Journal of Experimental Medicine. 2004;**200**(4):507-517. DOI: 10.1084/jem.20040590

[55] Moore ML, Newcomb DC, Parekh VV, Van Kaer L, Collins RD, Zhou W, et al. STAT1 negatively regulates lung basophil IL-4 expression induced by respiratory syncytial virus infection. Journal of Immunology (Baltimore, Md. 1950). 2009;**183**(3):2016-2026. DOI: 10.4049/jimmunol.0803167

[56] Parker EL, Silverstein RB, Verma S, Mysorekar IU. Viral-immune cell interactions at the maternal-fetal interface in human pregnancy. Frontiers in Immunology. 2020;**11**:522047. DOI: 10.3389/fimmu.2020.522047

[57] Eberlein B. Basophil activation as marker of clinically relevant allergy and therapy outcome. Frontiers in Immunology. 2020;**11**:1815. DOI: 10.3389/fimmu.2020.01815

[58] Hoarau JJ, Jaffar Bandjee MC, Krejbich Trotot P, Das T, Li-Pat-Yuen G, Dassa B, et al. Persistent chronic inflammation and infection by chikungunya arthritogenic alphavirus in spite of a robust host immune response. Journal of Immunology (Baltimore, Md.: 1950). 2010;**184**(10):5914-5927. DOI: 10.4049/jimmunol.0900255

[59] Pan J, Zhang M, Wang J, Wang Q, Xia D, Sun W, et al. Interferon-gamma is an autocrine mediator for dendritic cell maturation. Immunology Letters. 2004;**94**(1-2):141-151. DOI: 10.1016/j.imlet.2004.05.003

[60] Suzukawa M, Iikura M, Koketsu R, Nagase H, Tamura C, Komiya A, et al. An IL-1 cytokine member, IL-33, induces human basophil activation via its ST2 receptor. Journal of Immunology (Baltimore, Md.: 1950). 2008;**181**(9):5981-5989. DOI: 10.4049/jimmunol.181.9.5981

[61] Gambardella AR, Poto R, Tirelli V, Schroeder JT, Marone G, Mattei F, et al. Differential effects of alarmins on human and mouse basophils. Frontiers in Immunology. 2022;**13**:894163. DOI: 10.3389/fimmu.2022.894163

[62] Gunji Y, Matsumura T, Karasawa T, Komada T, Baatarjav C, Komori S, et al. IL-33-primed NLRP3 inflammasome in basophils drives IL-1β production and initiates atopic dermatitis inflammation. Cell death discovery, 2025;**11**(1):346. DOI: 10.1038/s41420-025-02630-6

[63] Zhu D, Kepley CL, Zhang M, Zhang K, Saxon A. A novel human immunoglobulin Fcγ–Fcε bifunctional fusion protein inhibits FcεRI-mediated degranulation. Nature Medicine. 2002;**8**(5):518-521. DOI: 10.1038/nm0502-518

[64] Cady CT, Powell MS, Harbeck RJ, Giclas PC, Murphy JR, Katial RK, et al. IgG antibodies produced during subcutaneous allergen immunotherapy mediate inhibition of basophil activation via a mechanism involving both FcgammaRIIA and FcgammaRIIB. Immunology Letters. 2010;**130**(1-2):57-65. DOI: 10.1016/j.imlet.2009.12.001

[65] Huang SU, O'Sullivan KM. The expanding role of extracellular traps in inflammation and autoimmunity: The new players in casting dark webs. International Journal of Molecular Sciences. 2022;**23**(7):3793. DOI: 10.3390/ijms23073793

Section 3

Eosinophils and Basophils in Cancer

Chapter 4

Perspective Chapter: Overview of Eosinophilia in Hematologic Cancers

Neslihan Mandacı Şanlı and Aysu Timuroğlu

Abstract

Eosinophils are bone marrow-derived cells involved in the regulation of the adaptive and innate immune system, tissue repair and remodeling. Eosinophils constitute 0.3–5% of leukocytes in the blood and are present in 50–500 per mm^3. If the absolute number of eosinophils in the blood is above $500/mm^3$, this is called eosinophilia. While eosinophilia frequently develops due to reactive (secondary) causes such as infection, allergy and drug reaction, primary eosinophilia is caused by malignant clones in myeloid/lymphoid neoplasms. Life-threatening organ damage may develop due to infiltration of tissues by eosinophils and release of granules. The differential diagnosis of eosinophilia is quite complex and requires a multidisciplinary approach. Eosinophilia may also be observed in hematologic malignancies, and it is an important condition that should be kept in mind in the differential diagnosis.

Keywords: eosinophilia, myeloid/lymphoid neoplasms with eosinophilia, tyrosine kinase, PDGFRA, hypereosinophilia

1. Introduction

Myeloid/lymphoid neoplasms with eosinophilia and PDGFRA, PDGFRB, FGFR1 and PCM1-JAK2 gene rearrangements are a relatively rare disease group. They were grouped under the heading "Myeloid/Lymphoid Neoplasms with Eosinophilia and Tyrosine Kinase Gene Fusions" in the 5th edition of the World Health Organization Classification of Hematolymphoid Tumors, published in 2022. This group of tumors is negative for the BCR-ABL1 gene transcript. These tumors have a variable clinical spectrum and respond well to tyrosine kinase inhibitor therapy. They can develop acutely or chronically and present in indolent or aggressive forms. They are a challenging group of diseases in which delays in diagnosis can occur, and morbidity/mortality can be high. In this article, we aimed to contribute to the literature by discussing these tumors in detail, along with their clinical findings and diagnostic stages [1–3].

2. Eosinophils and their biology and functions

Eosinophils are granulocytes originating from myeloid stem cells, containing dense cytoplasmic granules, showing intense avidity against the synthetic acid red dye "Eosin." The mature form of eosinophils, which are found very rarely in bone marrow and blood, is found in the gastrointestinal system (except the esophagus), lymphoid tissues, uterus and breast (**Figure 1**). Eosinophils synthesize numerous growth factors and cytokines and play a role in many homeostatic processes and inflammatory states [4]. They play an immune modulatory role in innate and adaptive immunity, have anti-inflammatory and anti-tumoral effects and are involved in tissue repair, remodeling, maintenance of tissue integrity and homeostasis [5]. In the bone marrow, cytokines such as interleukin-3 (IL-3), interleukin-5 (IL-5), granulocyte-macrophage colony stimulating factor (GM-CSF) and interleukin-33 (IL-33) enable the differentiation of myeloid precursor cells into eosinophils [1]. Eosinophils remain in the circulation for 25 hours before migrating to tissues [6].

Eosinophils have granules called major basic protein (MBP), eosinophil cationic protein (ECP), eosinophil peroxidase (EPO) and eosinophil-derived neurotoxin (EDN), and these granules cause tissue damage and dysfunction [4, 7–11]. ECPs are especially toxic to parasites and are also effective in bacterial, fungal and viral infections [2]. Although the role of eosinophils, which are involved in uterine maturation, in implantation and pregnancy has not yet been proven, it is known that eosinophils ectopically produce MBP in placental X and giant cells during pregnancy [12].

Eosinophils are typically seen in peripheral blood smears as cells measuring 14–16 microns in diameter, with a bilobed nucleus and pink-orange granules in the cytoplasm. In the flow cytometric examination, they are recognized by the expression of cd 45, cd15, cd66b, EMR-1, Siglec-8, CCR3[cd193], cd11b, cd13 and cd33 as surface antigens. Some clues can be used to differentiate morphologically normal eosinophils from reactive/malignant ones. Features such as loss of lobulation, hypersegmentation, cytoplasmic vacuoles and increased thickness of granules are mostly observed in malignant eosinophilia [2, 13, 14].

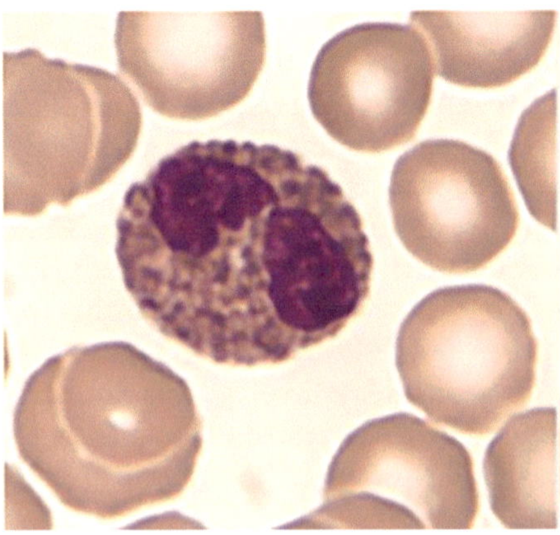

Figure 1.
Eosinophil in the peripheral blood smear [2]: Eosinophils have purple-violet colored granules and bilobed nucleus.

3. Eosinophilia

The number of eosinophils in peripheral blood is normal up to 500 cells per microliter (0.05–0.5 × 109/l) [15–17]. Eosinophils are the cells that are mostly localized in tissues due to the effects of eotaxins and chemokines and are found very rarely in peripheral blood. Eosinophilia can occur due to many causes, including allergic, inflammatory and neoplastic diseases, and requires a detailed examination. Eosinophilia is divided into three categories according to severity: mild (AEC: 0.5–1.49 × 109/l), moderate (1.5–5.0 × 109) and severe (>5.0 × 109/l). In peripheral blood, the eosinophil count is normal up to 500 cells per microliter (0.05–0.5 × 109/l), and AEC is measured in healthy volunteers and in patients with eosinophilic disease. Hypereosinophilia is the eosinophil count of 1500 or more cells per microliter (≥1.5 × 109/l); the causes of hypereosinophilia can be categorized into four titles as primary (clonal or neoplastic), secondary (reactive), hereditary (familial) and hypereosinophilia of undetermined significance [18–21]. Hypereosinophilia and hypereosinophilic syndromes are two different conditions. Hypereosinophilia is the presence of ≥1500 eosinophils per microliter with or without end-organ damage. In hypereosinophilic syndrome, there is eosinophilia-related organ dysfunction, accompanying an eosinophil count of ≥1500 per microliter (at least two measurements with an interval of ≥1 month) [20]. The term hypereosinophilic syndrome (HES) was first described by Hardy and Anderson in 1968 and defined as infiltration of organs, such as lung, heart and liver, by eosinophils for an unknown reason [22, 23]. The diagnosis of hypereosinophilic syndrome can be made in the absence of clonal eosinophilia, with persistent eosinophilia, exclusion of secondary causes and the presence of eosinophilia-related end-organ damage [20].

Although a peripheral blood count >5% is considered eosinophilia, it is more appropriate and accurate to use AEC when referring to eosinophilia. Because the percentage of eosinophils is affected by the white blood cell count and the distribution of leukocyte subtypes, in a normocellular bone marrow aspirate, >6% eosinophils are considered eosinophilia [18–20, 24, 25].

In clinical practice, the causes of eosinophilia are often secondary (reactive), and clonal eosinophilia is very rare. There are many causes of reactive eosinophilia, such as asthma, infections, drugs and solid organ tumors (**Table 1**). The eosinophilic disease can be corrected with the detection and treatment of the underlying clinical conditions. In particular, solid organ tumors can cause leukemoid reaction in the blood and hyperplasia in the bone marrow, leading to clinical findings very similar to that of myeloproliferative neoplasms. Occasionally, some hematologic neoplasms may also cause secondary eosinophilia with the release of eosinophilopoietic cytokines and may be a non-clonal cause of eosinophilia. The patient's history, clinical presentation and some specific tests are performed to determine the cause of eosinophilia and treatment targets, and agents are determined according to the underlying cause. The presence of clonality should be investigated and excluded by methods such as family history, peripheral blood and bone marrow examination, flow cytometric examination, histopathology, cytogenetics/fluorescence in situ hybridization (FISH) and polymerase chain reaction (PCR) [26–28].

In a patient presenting with eosinophilia, it is first necessary to exclude secondary causes and to determine if there are any end-organ related findings. A detailed travel history may be helpful in terms of parasitic infections. A stool examination for the detection of parasites or their eggs, and serum antibody tests are simple tests to be

Reactive [Secondary]
Infections:
Viral: HIV
Parasitic: echinococcus, entamoeba, toxocara, strongyloides, etc.
Bacterial: borreliosis, tuberculosis
Fungal: coccidioides, cryptococcus, pneumocystis, histoplasma
Drugs:
Non-steroidal anti-inflammatory drugs, aspirin
Allergic:
Asthma, Allergic rhinitis, atopic dermatitis, etc.
Autoimmune:
Eosinophilic granulomatosis with polyangiitis, immunoglobulin G4-related disease, diffuse fasciitis with eosinophilia, inflammatory bowel disease, celiac disease, rheumatoid arthritis
Malignancy:
Solid organ tumors, Hodgkin lymphoma, non-Hodgkin lymphoma
Metabolic:
Adrenal insufficiency
Immunodeficiency:
Hyper IgE syndromes, Wiskott-Aldrich syndrome
Others:
Acute/chronic graft versus host disease, solid organ rejection, cholesterol emboli, Gleich syndrome, and Kimura's disease
Clonal [Primary]
Myeloid/Lymphoid Neoplasms with Eosinophilia and Tyrosine Kinase Gene Fusions
Myeloid/lymphoid neoplasm with PDGFRA rearrangement
Myeloid/lymphoid neoplasm with PDGFRB rearrangement
Myeloid/lymphoid neoplasm with FGFR1 gene rearrangement
Myeloid/lymphoid neoplasm with PCM1:JAK2 gene rearrangement
Myeloid/lymphoid neoplasm with FLT3 gene rearrangement
Myeloid/lymphoid neoplasm with ETV6:ABL1 gene rearrangement
M/LN with eosinophilia and other alterations involving TK genes
Core Binding Factor Acute Myeloid Leukemia
Mastocytosis
Myeloproliferative Neoplasms
CML
CEL
Myelodysplastic/myeloproliferative neoplasms

Table 1.
Causes of eosinophilia.

performed as the first step in patients with eosinophilia. A detailed anamnesis should be taken regarding allergic diseases, collagen vascular diseases, gastrointestinal system and drug use. A detailed physical examination should be performed for palpable lymph nodes, splenomegaly and organomegaly.

Increased IgE levels are a nonspecific finding and are frequently seen in reactive states, but may sometimes be seen in primary HES Not Otherwise Specified (NOS) states. Similarly, increased haptocorrin production and therefore high vitamin B12 levels are among the expected findings in primary HES, NOS [29–31]. In patients with pulmonary symptoms, the presence of fibrosis may be investigated by lung tomography, chest radiography and bronchoscopy. Bronchoalveolar lavage and biopsy may be performed to investigate vasculitis, malignancy, etc. Troponin T and I, proBNP levels, echocardiography and electrocardiogram are useful tests in the detection of cardiac organ damage [1]. PET-CT is also one of the important imaging modalities that can be utilized while investigating eosinophilia (to rule out malignancy).

After the tests for secondary causes are performed and excluded, another test to be performed is bone marrow examination. Bone marrow biopsy is performed, and additional cytogenetic tests, including platelet-derived growth factor alpha (PDGFR-α), platelet-derived growth factor beta (PDGFR-ß), JAK2, t[9:22], fibroblast growth factor 1 (FGFR1), FMS-like tyrosine kinase (FLT3), STAT5B N642H mutation, etc., are studied from bone marrow aspirate/peripheral blood by FISH and PCR. Bone marrow biopsy evaluates the presence of dysplasia, myeloproliferation findings, presence of increased blasts, presence and degree of fibrosis and immunohistochemical staining for cd125, cd117, tryptase, etc. If no cause is found as a result of detailed investigations, a diagnosis of idiopathic hypereosinophilia is made, and if there is hypereosinophilia of undetermined significance or end-organ damage, a diagnosis of idiopathic HES is made [1].

4. Eosinophilia-associated hematologic malignancies

Eosinophilia may be seen in hematologic malignancies. Secondary (reactive) eosinophilia associated with eosinophilopoietic cytokine production is observed, especially in patients with lymphoid hematologic malignancies, whereas clonal (primary) eosinophilia originating from the malignant clone is frequently observed in myeloid hematologic neoplasms [2].

4.1 Primary (clonal) eosinophilia associated with hematologic malignancies

4.1.1 Myeloid/lymphoid neoplasms with eosinophilia and tyrosine kinase gene fusions (M/LN-eo-TK)

Myeloid or lymphoid neoplasms result from rearrangements involving genes that encode specific tyrosine kinases. This genetic rearrangement results in constitutive activation of the kinase domain and dysregulation of cell signaling pathways, leading to cell proliferation. In these neoplasms, the BCR/ABL1 gene transcript product is typically negative, and abnormal tyrosine kinase activation occurs as a result of the expression of fusion genes, including PDGFRA, PDGFRB, FGFR1, JAK2, FLT3 and other kinases. The resulting clinical picture has a very good response to TK inhibitor treatment (**Table 2**) [1, 2, 32–34]. These hematologic neoplasms have some common features: 1. There is a continuous activation of the tyrosine kinase signaling pathway as a result of gene fusion. 2. They can differentiate into myeloid and lymphoid

TK gene	Rearranged chromosomal band	Preferred TK inhibitor
PDGFRA	4q12	İmatinib
PDGFRB	5q32	İmatinib
FGFR1	t[8;13] [p11.2q12]	Ponatinib, sorafenib, pemigatinib, olverembatinib
PCM1:JAK2	t[8;9] [p22;p24]	Ruxolitinib, fedratinib
FLT3	t[12;13] [p13;q12]	Midostaurin, sorafenib, sunitinib, gilteritinib
ETV6:ABL1	t[9;12] [q34.1;p13.2]	İmatinib

Table 2.
Tyrosine kinase (TK) fusion genes associated with M/LN-eo and the tyrosine kinase inhibitor preferred.

progenitors as a result of mutation in bone marrow-derived stem cells and have complex and heterogeneous clinical manifestations. 3. Eosinophilia in bone marrow and peripheral blood is frequently associated. 4. They show excellent response to tyrosine kinase inhibitor therapy [35]. They can be diagnosed as myeloproliferative neoplasm (MPN), B/T acute lymphoblastic leukemia (ALL), myelodysplastic syndrome (MDS), MDS/MPN or acute myeloid leukemia (AML). Clinical manifestations are variable, with eosinophilia being the most common; extramedullary disease is also a common finding. The estimated incidence is <1/100,000 and is much rarer in children, with only a few cases reported [35]. It may have a chronic or acute, aggressive or indolent course. Hepatosplenomegaly, lymphadenopathy and constitutional symptoms may be observed. In some cases, chronic progression in the bone marrow may be accompanied by extramedullary involvement with an aggressive course [1, 2, 21, 32–34]. The category of M/LN-eo-TK contains several specific disease groups (PDGFRA, PDGFRB and FGFR1) and was recently expanded with JAK2-rearrangement (formerly a provisional entity), FLT3-rearrangements and ETV6::ABL1 in the 5th edition of the WHO classification (WHO-HAEM5) and the International Consensus Classification (ICC) [34, 36].

4.1.1.1 Myeloid/lymphoid neoplasm with PDGFRA rearrangement

PDGFRA gene, located in the 4q12 region, is involved in encoding the synthesis of a TK receptor protein involved in cell survival, division and proliferation. Myeloid/lymphoid neoplasm with PDGFRA rearrangement is the most common form of M/LN-eo and is most commonly seen in males (M/F:16/1), with female and pediatric cases rarely reported. It occurs in the late 40s (20–50 years). Fatigue, pruritus, dyspnea and cough are the common symptoms, and restrictive or obstructive lung disease, endomyocardial fibrosis, Loeffler's endocarditis and valvular regurgitation can be seen [37]. In patients with PDGFRA gene rearrangement, eosinophilia is seen in the bone marrow and peripheral blood. Like in chronic eosinophilic leukemia (CEL), extramedullary tumors are present in 50% of cases, and extramedullary involvement alone, without bone marrow involvement, is rarely seen. Cases with normal eosinophil values have also been reported. Serum vitamin b12 and tryptase levels may be measured high [35, 38, 39]. Bone marrow is frequently hypercellular; eosinophil precursors are increased, eosinophils are dysmorphic and normal morphology. Blast rate is <20%. Increased mast cells can be seen in clusters, and they are frequently cd25 positive. Moderate fibrosis can be observed [38–40]. Rarely, the disease in this indolent clinical form may transform into a blastic aggressive form, T/B-ALL, or may be transformed into AML [41]. Much fewer cases may present as AML with eosinophilia. In the literature, a case of T-cell cutaneous lymphoma with FIP1L1:PDGFRA rearrangement accompanied by three synchronous hematologic malignancies, T lymphoblastic leukemia in the lymph node and MPN in the bone marrow, has been reported [42].

In cases with PDGFRA gene rearrangement, the most common gene partner is FIP1L1. There is an interstitial cryptic deletion at 4q12, resulting in FIP1L1:PDGFRA gene fusion (in 85% of cases), while different fusions of PDGFR occur in some cases [34, 43–45]. KIF5B, CDK5RAP2, STRN, ETV6, BCR, TNKS2 and FOX1 are other partner genes that make variant translocations with PDGFRA [2]. In the presence of marked eosinophilia in the tissue or subsequent development of myeloid neoplasia, the presence of PDGFRA should be investigated by FISH or real-time (RT) PCR (**Figure 2**). Both peripheral blood and bone marrow samples are sufficient for genetic

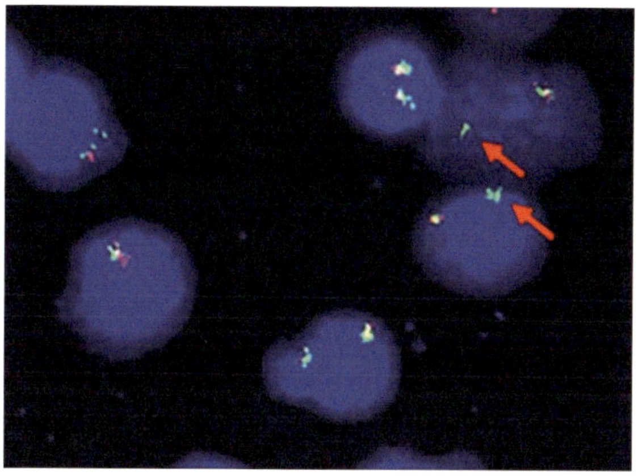

Figure 2.
PDGFRA gene rearrangement showed with FISH [41]: By fluorescence in situ hybridization rearrranged PDGFRA gene [arrows]. Rearrengements results from fusion of FIPL1 and PDGFRA.

analysis. RT-PCR can detect PDGFRA and FIP1L1 gene rearrangement, but not other gene partners. Next-generation sequencing (NGS) can also be performed. However, if molecular diagnosis is not possible, this diagnosis may be suspected in the presence of Philadelphia (Ph) chromosome-negative MPN and clinical findings resembling chronic eosinophilic leukemia, increased mast cell count, increased mast cell tryptase level, splenomegaly and high serum vitamin B12 levels [2, 35, 39].

All cases with PDGFRA gene rearrangements respond to imatinib and are more than 100 times more sensitive than BCR:ABL1. The dose of imatinib in patients in the chronic phase is 100 mg/day, with concomitant corticosteroids recommended in patients with cardiac involvement. In patients in the blastic phase, imatinib 100–400 mg/day is used concurrently with chemotherapy [2, 39].

4.1.1.2 Myeloid/lymphoid neoplasm with PDGFRB rearrangement

PDGFRB gene, located at 5q32, encodes a TK receptor protein involved in mitogenic activity in mesenchymal cells [2]. The male/female incidence rate is 2/1, and it is observed frequently in the late 40s. Its incidence constitutes <2% of all MPNs. In 50–85% cases, hypereosinophilia is seen, while in 21–25% cases, monocytosis is more prominent while eosinophilia is absent. Anemia and thrombocytopenia are also expected findings in these patients [35, 37, 39, 46, 47]. Bone marrow examination may show CMML, atypical CM, AML, de novo B-ALL and T-ALL/LBL. There is a hypercellular bone marrow due to neutrophilic and eosinophilic infiltration. Mast cells may also be seen, and fibrosis may be present. The most commonly involved organ is spleen (83%); hepatomegaly may accompany end-organ damage associated with eosinophilia. Skin findings are very rare. Serum tryptase levels may increase [35, 37, 39, 47].

In cases with PDGFRB rearrangement, ETV6:PDFGRB is often caused by t[5;12][q32;p13.2]. More than 40 different gene partners have been identified, and ETV6 is the most common. In addition to ETV6-PDGFRB gene rearrangement, de novo B-ALL associated with EBF1, EBF1, SSBP2, TNIP1, ZEB2 and ATF7IP (partner genes), Ph-like B-ALL cases can be seen. Increasingly, cryptic translocations have been identified, and therefore, in cases where peripheral blood or bone marrow eosinophilia cannot be explained, such as inversion 16, PDGFRB gene rearrangements should be investigated for the presence of PDGFRB gene rearrangements [2, 3, 21, 48–50]. Genetic analysis can be performed from bone marrow or peripheral blood [51]. In addition, in the presence of eosinophilia accompanying morphologically or immunophenotypically abnormal mast cells, the presence of PDGFRB should be investigated by FISH if there is no KIT mutation. RT-PCR can detect a very small number of PDGFRB-associated clones and is useless except for PDGFRB-ETV6, while FISH can detect all PDGFRB rearrangements but not partner genes. Importantly, t[5:12] and other PDGFRB fusions can also be seen in BCR-ABL1-like B-ALL [3, 18, 35, 39, 48, 52–54].

It is recommended to use imatinib 400 mg/day in chronic-phase patients and concurrent chemotherapy in blastic-phase patients. Nearly 100% complete hematologic response (CHR) and up to 86% complete cytogenetic remission (CCR) can be achieved, and after CHR and CCR are achieved, it may be considered to reduce the imatinib dose to 100 mg/day [39].

4.1.1.3 Myeloid/lymphoid neoplasm with FGFR1 gene rearrangement

FGFR1 gene is localized at 8p11 and is involved in the synthesis of TK receptor protein involved in cell maturation, development and mitosis. They are recognized by the presence of fusion genes arising from t[8;13][p11.2q12] or variant translocations [2, 18, 55]. They are rare and are reported as case series in the literature (<1% of all MPN cases) [39, 56]. It is a heterogeneous group of diseases, with a male/female ratio of 1.5/1 and is more common in the 30s. Interestingly, this disease is also seen in children and the elderly [39, 55, 57]. Cases with FGFR1 gene rearrangement present as eosinophilia-related chronic myeloid neoplasia or blastic-phase disease with B-cell, T-cell, myeloid or mixed phenotypic origin [34]. In some cases, genetic abnormalities may occur during the clinical course of MDS or MDS/MPN or during the transformation of MPN into blastic phase [2].

Cytogenetically, the most frequent translocation is t[8;13][p11;q12] or ZNF198::FGFR1 (41–48%), followed by t[8;22][p11.2;q11.2]/BCR::FGFR1 [18–29%], t[8;9][p12;q33]/CEP110::FGFR1 [12–17%] and t[6;8][q27;p11.2]/FGFR1OP::FGFR1 (9–12%); other variant translocations or insertions are uncommon. These cytogenetic abnormalities can be detected using FISH or RT-PCR. While some cases may present with monocytosis and tonsillar hypertrophy, others may present with monocytosis and B-ALL [35]. Constitutive symptoms, lymphadenopathy and eosinophilia may be observed. Hepatosplenomegaly, neutrophilia and monocytosis are expected findings [39, 58–60].

FGFR1-rearranged neoplasms are usually not responsive to imatinib or second-generation tyrosine kinase inhibitör (TKI). The presence of RUNX1 mutations and unresponsiveness to TKI treatment are associated with poor prognosis, and allogeneic hematopoietic stem cell transplantation (ASCT) may be effective in disease control in selected cases [35, 58, 60]. In case series published in recent years, treatment agents such as ponatinib, sorafenib, pemigatinib and olverembatinib have been reported to be effective [55, 61–64].

4.1.1.4 Myeloid/lymphoid neoplasm with PCM1:JAK2 gene rearrangement

The JAK2 gene is localized at 9p24 and is involved in the synthesis of a TK protein responsible for cell proliferation. M/LN-eo with t[8;9][p22;p24]/PCM::JAK2 and its genetic variants (involving 9p24/JAK2) cause a wide clinical spectrum of diseases with diverse molecular genetic features and several co-mutations [2, 35]. JAK2 V617 mutation has been demonstrated in many myeloproliferative neoplasms, but JAK2 gene-related translocations are observed in very few hematologic cancers, with t[8;9][p22;p24] being the most common. It was first described in 1990 in philadelphia chromosome (Ph)-negative neutrophilic myelofibrosis. This gene rearrangement affects numerous hematopoietic lineages and can be found in chronic- or blastic-phase hematologic neoplasms accompanied by eosinophils [2, 65]. JAK2 may also rearrange with ETV6 or BCR, and somatic mutations may also be observed [35, 66]. FISH or RT-PCR can be used to confirm JAK2-related translocations [39].

To date, about 100 cases associated with t[8;9][p22;p24] and its variants have been reported and it is predominantly male dominant (male/female ratio: 3/4), and the age of onset is quite wide with the most common age range being late 40s [51, 67–73]. Chronic MPN with increased eosinophilia, immature erythroid progenitors and bone marrow fibrosis is the most common presentation of MDS/MPN; however, to a lesser extent, it can also present as MDS, AML, de novo B/T-ALL or lymphoblastic crisis of myeloproliferative disorders, and cutaneous T-cell lymphoma. Interestingly, those with de novo B-ALL in this group do not have eosinophilia in the bone marrow or peripheral blood, and a differential diagnosis with Ph-like B-ALL is essential in these cases because Ph-like B-ALL also has JAK2 gene rearrangements. Especially, the presence of rearrangements with gene partners such as SSBP2, PAX5, RFX3, USP25 and ZNF274 supports the diagnosis of Ph-like B-ALL [3, 68, 72, 74–77]. Extramedullary involvement is common. Lymphadenopathy may also be observed. Overall survival is variable, and especially blastic phases have a very poor prognosis [2, 33, 73, 74, 76, 78]. Patients in the chronic phase may be given ruxolitinib or fedratinib, while in the blastic phase, TKIs are recommended in combination with chemotherapy. Imatinib, dasatinib and nilotinib are not effective, and ASCT is the only curative treatment option [35, 39].

4.1.1.5 Myeloid/lymphoid neoplasm with FLT3 gene rearrangement

FTL3 is a type 3 class 3 TK receptor involved in cell proliferation, survival, differentiation and regulation. M/LN-eo-TK with FLT3 gene rearrangement has been identified as a new group in WHO-HAEM5 and ICC. ETV6 fusion occurs as a result of t[12;13][p13;q12]. It is an extremely rare group of diseases with about 35 cases described in the literature, with clinical presentation as CEL, T-LBL or peripheral T-cell lymphoma. Similar to atypical CML, JMML and systemic mastocytosis, it may also present as MDS/MPN or MPN (**Figure 3**). Extramedullary involvement is frequent, occurs mostly in blastic cases and has a very aggressive course [2, 34–36, 39]. Although ETV6 is the most common gene partner, ZMYM2, TRIP11, SPTBN1, GOLGB1, CCDC88C, MYO18A and BCR are other partner genes and somatic mutations may also be present. It has a wide age range and is more common in males than females. There is eosinophilia in tissues, blood and bone marrow [79, 80]. Cases may respond to FLT3 inhibitors (midostaurin, sorafenib, sunitinib and gilteritinib) and ASCT in some patients [2, 39].

4.1.1.6 Myeloid/lymphoid neoplasm with ETV6:ABL1 gene rearrangement

ABL1 gene is localized on the ninth chromosome and encodes a TK protein involved in the regulation of cell proliferation and apoptosis, myeloid/lymphoid

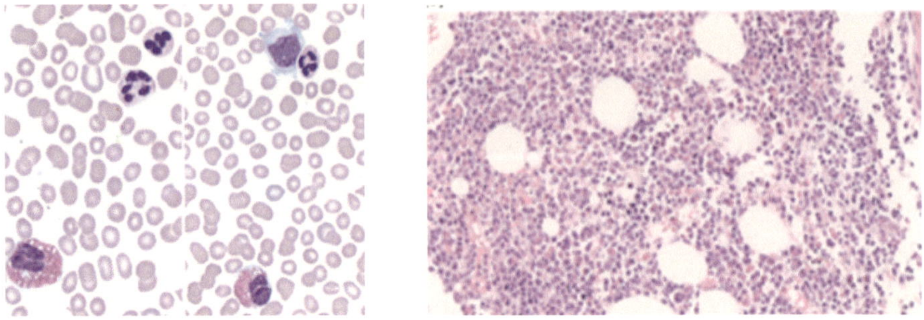

Figure 3.
M/LN with Flt3 fusion presenting as B-LBL [35]: Peripheral blood smear and bone marrow biopsy figures of a patient diagnosed as M/LN neoplasm with flt3 fusion presenting as B-LBL. In the left picture, there are dysplastic neutrophils and eosinophilia at the peripheral blood smear. The right one is a figure of bone marrow biopsy: hypercellular with increased blasts, spindle-shaped mast cells and eosinophilia.

neoplasm with t[9;12] [q34.1;p13.2]/ETV6: The only gene partner of BL1 gene in ABL1 cases is ETV6. Chronic myeloid leukemia with eosinophilia presents as a group of diseases with clinical and laboratory findings similar to CMML, and in the presence of this gene rearrangement, it may also present as MPN, B- and T-box lymphoblastic leukemia or AML cases. More than 13 gene partners of ABL1 have been identified in de novo T-ALL cases and PH-like B-ALL cases [2, 81–86]. When we look at the pathogenesis of these diseases, we see that they occur as a result of ETV6 insertion into ABL1 or ABL1 insertion into ETV6, rather than t[9;12]. ETV6/ABL1 gene fusion is very difficult to detect; karyotyping may be inadequate and FISH may miss cryptic translocations with false negatives because they are very small insertions and may not produce a visible cleavage signal. Therefore, RT-PCR using specific probes targeting ETV6 and ABL1 can detect this molecular alteration. RNA sequencing is also a preferable method to confirm this gene rearrangement [2, 35].

If we look at the clinical presentation of hematologic neoplasms with ETV6:ABL1 gene rearrangement, ETV6:ABL1 shows a tyrosine kinase activity similar to BCR:ABL1; therefore, the cases have very similar clinical features to chronic myeloid leukemia. Chronic-phase CML has very similar morphologic findings; eosinophilia and basophilia are expected findings. These patients may have blastic transformation like CML cases, and especially B-ALL cases have very similar clinical features to Ph-like B-ALL cases. The number of cases with myeloid/lymphoid neoplasm with ETV6:ABL1 gene rearrangement is about 60, and male gender is dominant in general (M/F Ratio: 3.5:1) [2, 35]. While patients in the chronic phase are responsive to tyrosine kinase inhibitor treatment, those in the blastic phase have a poor prognosis and poor response to TKI treatment [2, 21, 35, 78, 86]. Patients in the blastic phase should be given chemotherapy together with TKI, and ASCT should be performed at the earliest period [39].

4.1.1.7 M/LN with eosinophilia and other alterations involving TK genes

M/LN with eosinophilia and genetic alterations, including ETV6::FGFR2, ETV6::LYN, ETV6::NTRK3, RANBP2::ALK, BCR::RET and FGFR1OP::RET, have been described, and they are very rare cases. It is thought that these cases may also be responsive to TKI treatment, but there is no complete clarity due to the small number of cases and experience [2, 35].

4.1.2 Core binding factor acute myeloid leukemia

Core binding factor (CBF) is a transcription factor with an important role in the regulation of normal hematopoiesis. CBF acute myeloid leukemias are leukemias with cytogenetically defined t[8;21][q22;q22] or inv[16][p13q22]/t[16;16][p13;q22] positivity. The rearrangements t[8;21] and inv[16] involve the RUNX1/RUNX1T1 (AML1-ETO) and CBFB/MYH11 genes, respectively. In the presence of these recurrent cytogenetic abnormalities, WHO defines acute myeloid leukemia regardless of the blast count, even if the blast count in bone marrow or peripheral blood is <20% [87, 88].

T[8;21][q22;q22] positive AML is mostly seen in young people and accounts for about 5% of all acute myeloid leukemia cases. Inversion 16 or t[16;16] positive AML is a clinical entity that can be observed in all age groups and accounts for 5–8% of all AML cases [89]. As in all cases of AML, cytopenias related with deterioration of hematopoiesis, bleeding, coagulopathy, diffuse bone pain or susceptibility to infections are common clinical findings in both. Extramedullary involvement is more common in iv 16/t[16;16]-positive AML cases compared to t[8;21] positive cases. It is frequently monocytic or myelomonocytic, and eosinophil levels in the blood are frequently normal [87, 90–93]. In some cases presenting with hyperleukocytosis, eosinophilia is observed and eosinophil morphology is frequently normal, but may also be dysplastic. In bone marrow examination, there is marked eosinophilia and immature eosinophilic cells are present [2, 87, 92, 93].

In t[8;21]-positive AML cases, blasts are characteristically quite large, with basophilic cytoplasm and large azurophilic granules. Blasts may have Pseudo-Chediak-Higashi granules or auer body. Normal eosinophils are present and can reach quite high numbers [89]. Marked eosinophilia may be observed in both the bone marrow and blood. In t[8;21]-positive AML cases, eosinophils often have normal cytologic morphology, whereas in inversion 16/t[16;16]-positive AML cases, all stages of eosinophilic maturation can be seen and immature eosinophilic cytoplasmic granules can be seen in promyelocyte and myelocyte stages. These immature eosinophilic granules are larger than normal and may be purple-violet in color (**Figure 4**). These abnormal eosinophils demonstrate faint positivity for the naphthol AS-D chloroacetate esterase reaction and PAS reaction, which is normally negative in eosinophils.

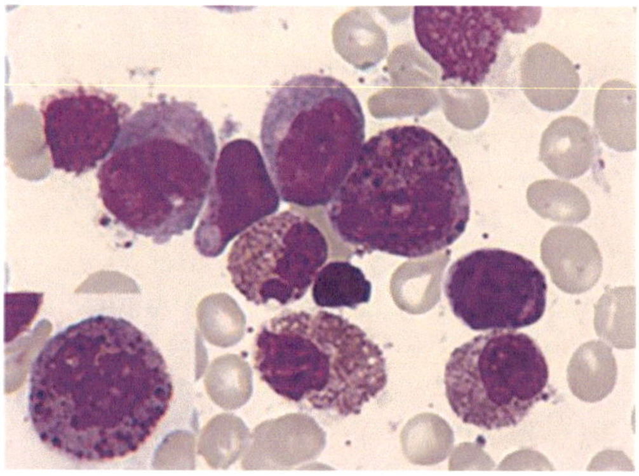

Figure 4.
Inversion 16 positive AML with eosinophilia [2]: A bone marrow aspirate of a patient with inversion 16 positive AML: there are dysplastic eosinophils with purple-violet granules.

In T [8;21]-positive AML cases, the chloroacetate reaction and PAS reaction may be negative/positive in eosinophils [2, 89, 92, 94, 95].

In order to diagnose CBF acute myeloid leukemia, cytogenetic, FISH or RT-PCR analysis should be performed to demonstrate molecular alterations. Also, FISH and PCR assays are useful to confirm that the rearrangements actually involve the RUNX1/RUNX1T1 (AML1-ETO) and CBFB/MYH11 genes in t[8;21] and inv[16], respectively, as inv[16] may be cryptic by conventional cytogenetics [96]. A recent striking feature is that KIT gene mutation may accompany these cases and its effect on prognosis. KIT gene encodes a tyrosine kinase receptor that plays an important role in cell proliferation and survival, and is found as an additional cytogenetic anomaly in 20–25% of t[8;21] positive cases and in 30% of inversion 16 positive cases [97, 98]. In general, CBF-positive AML cases are included in the good prognostic group in the European LeukemiaNet (ELN) 2022 guidelines and have good response rates with standard AML therapy. However, of course, the presence of additional cytogenetic abnormalities may negatively affect the prognosis; for example, KIT gene mutation is associated with a high risk of relapse, while deletion [9q] is an unfavorable prognostic criterion [91, 97, 99].

4.1.3 Mastocytosis

Mastocytosis is a rare systemic/localized disease with a prevalence of 1 in 10,000. It is seen at similar rates in both sexes. Systemic involvement is often encountered in patients diagnosed in adulthood and is permanent, whereas >90% of mastocytosis in childhood is limited to skin involvement and findings resolve by adulthood [100–102]. Systemic mastocytosis (SM) is a clonal disease of mast cells and presents with splenomegaly, skin involvement, gastrointestinal system involvement, etc., and a very small proportion of cases present with eosinophilia [37].

Although the basic pathological disorder in mastocytosis is not fully understood, stem cell factor (SCF), also known as c-kit ligand, is required for mast cell formation and development from hematopoietic progenitor cells, and SCF receptors are located on the mast cell surface. This receptor is the TK-KIT receptor (cd117), and genetic mutations in KIT or in the gene encoding KIT in patients with mastocytosis may cause SCF overexpression and lead to mastocytosis clinic. Anaphylaxis and allergic reactions occur as a result of sudden and intense release of these mediators by mast cells containing a large number of vasoactive mediators [103–105]. In addition, urticaria pigmentosa, splenomegaly, hepatomegaly, pathologic bone fractures, abdominal pain, food allergy, etc. may also be observed [106–111].

Systemic mastocytosis may be associated with a hematologic neoplasm. These cases are frequently diagnosed in the sixth decade. Skin involvement and symptoms related to mediator release are less common compared to indolent mastocytosis types, while splenomegaly, lymphadenopathy, hepatomegaly and constitutional symptoms are more common. In up to 90% of cases, the accompanying hematologic neoplasm is of myeloid origin [112, 113]. Rarely, a lymphoproliferative disease such as acute myeloid leukemia, non-Hodgkin's and Hodgkin's lymphoma, or multiple myeloma may be observed [114, 115].

Peripheral eosinophilia may be observed in 28% of patients with systemic mastocytosis, and this frequency may increase even more in advanced forms of mastocytosis [116, 117]. Eosinophilia may be found in bone marrow biopsy or aspiration samples of patients who do not have significant eosinophilia in the peripheral blood [118, 119]. Mastocytosis should be considered especially in the presence of findings, such as organomegaly, elevated vitamin B12, eosinophilia, anemia and thrombocytopenia. M/LN-eo group diseases must be excluded in these patients; patients with mastocytosis have cd 25 and cd 2 expression, whereas M/LN-eo group diseases may have mast cell increase and aberrant expression of cd 25 but not cd 2 expression. KIT mutation is not found in M/LN-eo group diseases. Another important feature in patients with systemic mastocytosis is cd 30 positivity on the mast cell surface in 80% cases and this is an important marker in differentiating from M/LN-eo group diseases [34, 120, 121].

4.1.4 Myeloproliferative neoplasms

Myeloproliferative neoplasms are a clonal group of diseases characterized by an increase in myeloid lineage cells in the peripheral blood. Although eosinophilia can be seen in all subtypes, it is most commonly seen in CML and chronic eosinophilic leukemia (CEL). The BCR:ABL1 gene fusion product resulting from t[9;22] [q34;q11] plays a role in the pathogenesis of CML, while many different somatic mutations such as JAK2 p.V617F, JAK2 exon 12, CALR and MPL play a role in others. In diseases other than CML, t[9;22] [q34;q11] is negative. This group of diseases, which frequently progress in the chronic phase, may also progress to blastic phase [34].

Patients with CML are often characterized by increased neutrophils and neutrophil precursor cells in the peripheral blood, and eosinophilia may also be present. The eosinophilic variant of CML is very rare and has a very poor prognosis. Fibrosis occurs as a result of the exposure of eosinophilic granules in the peripheral blood due to eosinophilia, and tissue damage is observed most commonly in the heart and lung [122].

In chronic myeloproliferative neoplasms, leukocytosis is associated with unfavorable clinical outcome, especially in polycythemia vera and essential thrombocytosis, and has been associated with decreased survival, risk of leukemic progression, disease progression and increased risk of thrombosis [123].

CEL is a myeloproliferative neoplasm characterized by increased eosinophils in the blood, bone marrow and peripheral tissues as a result of proliferation of eosinophilic precursors. It is frequently confused with hypereosinophilic syndrome. The age of onset is the fourth decade of life, and it is more common in males. CEL diagnostic criteria: 1. Persistent eosinophilia $\geq$1.5 × 109/L in the blood, increased bone marrow eosinophils; 2. > 5% but >19% myeloblasts in the bone marrow or > 2% in the peripheral blood; 3.Clonality of myeloid cells; 4. No reactive eosinophilia due to allergy, parasitic, infectious, pulmonary or collagen vascular disease; 5. No reactive eosinophilia due to other malignancies [124]. It may be confused with CEL/hypereosinophilic syndrome. The absence of genetic clonality, blast increase or abnormal morphology in the bone marrow suggests the diagnosis of hypereosinophilic syndrome [2]. In CEL, fibrosis-related damage is most commonly seen in the lung and heart. Hepatomegaly and splenomegaly are expected findings. Dysplasia may be seen in eosinophils, including cytoplasmic vacuolization, three-lobed nucleus or ring formation in the nucleus. Hyper/hypogranulation may be seen in eosinophils. Microeosinophils may also be seen. Some eosinophils may show both eosinophilic and basophilic granulation. Fibrosis may be observed in the bone marrow, and it is characterized with leukocytosis in the peripheral blood [124, 125].

4.1.5 Myelodysplastic/myeloproliferative neoplasms

Myelodysplastic/myeloproliferative neoplasms are a heterogeneous group of hematologic neoplasms and are overlap syndromes with both dysplastic and myeloproliferative features; eosinophilia may also be observed in these diseases. They may have a chronic, slow course or aggressive form showing transformation into acute leukemia. Rarely, they may present with eosinophilia, originating from the malignant clone. Nevertheless, in the presence of eosinophilia in a patient with MDS, secondary causes should be investigated and excluded.

4.2 Reactive eosinophilia in hematologic neoplasms

4.2.1 Lymphoid neoplasms

Eosinophilia may be seen at the time of diagnosis or after chemotherapy in both B- and T-cell leukemias and lymphomas. However, eosinophilia is more common in T-cell lymphoid malignancies than in B-cell lymphoid malignancies, especially in Hodgkin's lymphoma and t[5;14] positive acute lymphoblastic leukemia.

4.2.2 T-cell lymphoid hematologic neoplasms

Adult T-cell leukemia/lymphoma and T-cell lymphoblastic lymphoma are hematologic neoplasms with peripheral eosinophilia, with rates up to 30%. Eosinophilia is observed especially as a result of the release of IL-5, GM-CSF and IL-3-like cytokines, which are eosinopoietic cytokines released from malignant T-cells [126, 127]. Eosinophilia in these malignancies is not clonal but rather originates from the inflammatory background around the tumor cells. Mycosis fungoides, cutaneous T-cell lymphoma and Sezary syndrome are also characterized by eosinophilia and an increase in IgE, with rates up to approximately 20%. The frequency of eosinophilia is higher in Sezary syndrome [128–130], while eosinophilia is observed in 32–50% of cases in the angioimmunoblastic type of nodal T-follicular helper cell lymphoma. Eosinophilia is rarely an expected finding in other T-cell lymphoma types [2].

4.2.3 B-cell lymphoid hematologic neoplasms

Eosinophilia in tissue is a common finding in Hodgkin's lymphoma and less common in B-cell non-Hodgkin's lymphoma. In Hodgkin's lymphoma, mild eosinophilia is seen in approximately 15% of cases and they mostly surround the inflammatory background around the histologically Reed-Sternberg cells. Again, t[5;14] [q31.1;q32.3/IL3::IGH] positive cases, which is a rare subtype of B-cell acute lymphoblastic leukemia, are also associated with reactive eosinophilia, and eosinophilia may be observed before clinical findings appear [2, 131, 132].

4.2.4 Lymphocytic variant of hypereosinophilic syndrome

It is a rare subtype of hypereosinophilic syndrome and is a variant with primarily skin and soft tissue involvement, cardiac, pulmonary and joint involvement. Eosinophilia may be observed due to the release of eosinophilopoietic cytokines from clonal T cells with abnormal immunophenotype. Serum IgE levels are frequently high. There is abnormal IL-5, IL-4, IL-13 and GM-CSF production from T cells. There is evidence of eosinophilia-related tissue and organ damage. Male-to-female ratios are similar, and it may evolve into lymphoma [2, 113, 133, 134]. Cutaneous lesions, erythroderma, angioedema, urticaria and polyclonal hypergammaglobulinemia may be observed clinically. There is no standard treatment, and corticosteroids, cyclophosphamide and methotrexate may be used [37].

5. Conclusion

Eosinophilia can cause fibrosis with a wide variety of causes, resulting in tissue/organ damage. In hematologic malignancies, eosinophilia can be clonal/reactive and the diagnosis requires very detailed investigations and genetic analysis. The diagnostic phase in a patient with eosinophilia is a long and difficult process and requires adequate molecular support, flow cytometric examination, bone marrow examination and detailed imaging studies. Hematologic malignancies associated with clonal eosinophilia are rare, and more clinical data and studies are needed. We believe that we will have more data in the future with the development of diagnostic tests and increased awareness.

Author details

Neslihan Mandacı Şanlı[1*] and Aysu Timuroğlu[2]

1 Department of Hematology, Erciyes University, Kayseri, Turkey

2 Department of Hematology, Erzurum City Hospital, Erzurum, Turkey

*Address all correspondence to: ortoforia@hotmail.com

References

[1] Schomali W, Gotlib J. In: Kaushansky K, Lichtman MA, Prchal JT, Levi M, Burns LJ, Linch DC, editors. Eosinophils and their Disorders. Wiiliams Hematology Tenth Edition. New York: Mc Graw Hill; 2021. pp. 1081-1092

[2] Morales-Camacho RM, Caballero-Velázquez T, Borrero JJ, et al. Hematological neoplasms with eosinophilia. Cancers. 2024;**16**(337):1-28

[3] Reiter A, Gotlib J. Myeloid neoplasms with eosinophilia. Blood. 2017;**129**(6):704-714

[4] Blanchard C, Rothenberg ME. Advances in Immunology. 2009;**101**:81-121

[5] Kanda A, Yasutaka Y, Van Bui D, et al. Multiple biological aspects of eosinophils in host defense, eosinophil-associated diseases, immunoregulation, and homeostasis: Is their role beneficial, detrimental, regulator, or bystander? Biological & Pharmaceutical Bulletin. 2020;**43**:20-23

[6] Farahi N, Singh NR, Heard S, et al. Use of 111-Indiium-labeled autologous eosinophils to establish the *in vivo* kinetics of human eosinophils In healthy subjects. Blood. 2012;**120**(19):4068-4071

[7] Gleich GJ, Adolphson CR. Advances in Immunology. 1986;**39**:177

[8] Gleich GJ, Frigas E, Loegering DA, et al. Journal of Immunology. 1979;**123**:2925

[9] Frigas E, Loegering DA, Gleich GJ. Laboratory Investigation. 1980;**42**:35

[10] Tai PC, Hayes DJ, Clark JB, et al. The Biochemical Journal. 1982;**204**:75

[11] Venge P, Dahl R, Hallgren R, et al. In: Mahmoud AAF, Austin KF, editors. The Eosinophil in Health and Disease. New York: Grune and Stratton; 1980. p. 1131

[12] Wagner JM, Hustin J, Bonno M, et al. Placenta. 1994;**15**:625

[13] Lee JJ, Jacobsen EA, Ochkur SI, et al. Human versus mouse eosinophils: 'That which we call an eosinophil, by any other name would stain As red'. The Journal of Allergy and Clinical Immunology. 2012;**130**(3):572-584

[14] Goasguen JE, Bennett JM, Bain BJ, et al. International working group on morphology of MDS. The role of eosinophil morphology in distinguishing between reactive eosinophilia and eosinophilia as a feature of a myeloid neoplasm. British Journal of Haematology. 2020;**191**:497-504

[15] Spector SL, Tan RA. Is a single blood eosinophil count a reliable marker for "eosinophilic asthma?". The Journal of Asthma. 2012;**49**:807

[16] Statland BE, Winkel P, Harris SC, et al. Evaluation of biologic sources of variation of leukocyte counts and other hematologic quantities using very precise automated analyzers. American Journal of Clinical Pathology. 1978;**69**:48

[17] Sennels HP, Jørgensen HL, Hansen AL, et al. Diurnal variation of hematology parameters in healthy young males: The Bispebjerg study of diurnal variations. Scandinavian Journal of Clinical and Laboratory Investigation. 2011;**71**:532

[18] Bain BJ. Eosinophilic leukaemias and the idiopathic hypereosinophilic

syndrome. British Journal of Haematology. 1996;**95**:2-9

[19] Valent P, Klion AD, Horny HP, et al. Contemporary consensus proposal on criteria and classification of eosinophilic disorders and related syndromes. The Journal of Allergy and Clinical Immunology. 2012;**130**:607-612.e9

[20] Valent P, Klion AD, Roufosse F, et al. Proposed refined diagnostic criteria and classification of eosinophil disorders and related syndromes. Allergy. 2023;**78**:47-59

[21] Shomali W, Gotlib J. World Health Organization-defined eosinophilic disorders: 2019 update on diagnosis, risk stratification, and management. American Journal of Hematology. 2019;**94**(10):1149-1167

[22] Hardy WR, Andersen RE. The hypereosinophilic syndromes. Annals of Internal Medicine. 1968;**68**(6):1220-1229

[23] Chusid MJ, Dale DC, West BC, et al. The hypereosinophilic syndrome: Analysis of fourteen cases with review of the literature. Medicine (Baltimore). 1975;**54**(1):1-27

[24] Tefferi A. Blood eosinophilia: A new paradigm in disease classification, diagnosis, and treatment. Mayo Clinic Proceedings. 2005;**80**:75

[25] Roufosse F, Weller PF. Practical approach to the patient with hypereosinophilia. The Journal of Allergy and Clinical Immunology. 2010;**126**:39

[26] Guenzel AJ, Smadbeck JB, Golden CL, et al. Clinical utility of next generation sequencing to detect IGH/IL3 rearrangements [t(5;14)(q31.1;q32.1)] in B-lymphoblastic leukemia/lymphoma. Annals of Diagnostic Pathology. 2021;**53**:151761

[27] Romagnoli S, Bartalucci N, Gesullo F, et al. Nanopore sequencing for the screening of myeloid and lymphoid neoplasms with eosinophilia and rearrangement of Pdgfrα, Pdgfrβ, FGFR1 or PCM1-JAK2. Biomarker Research. 2021;**9**:83

[28] Podvin B, Roynard P, Boudry A, et al. Whole-genome optical mapping to elucidate myeloid/lymphoid neoplasms with eosinophilia and tyrosine kinase gene fusions. Leukemia Research. 2022;**123**:106972

[29] Ogbogu PU, Bochner BS, Butterfield JH, et al. Hypereosinophilic syndrome: A multicenter, retrospective analysis of clinical characteristics and response to therapy. The Journal of Allergy and Clinical Immunology. 2009;**124**(6):1319-1325

[30] Helbig G, Soja A, Bartkowska-Chrobok A, et al. Chronic eosinophilic leukemia-not otherwise specified has a poor prognosis with unresponsiveness to conventional treatment and high risk of a transformation. American Journal of Hematology. 2012;**87**(6):643-645

[31] Andres E, Serraj K, Zhu J, et al. The pathophysiology of elevated vitamin B12 in clinical practise. QJM. 2013;**106**(6):505-515

[32] Kim AS, Pozdnyakova O. SOHO state of the art updates and next questions|myeloid/lymphoid neoplasms with eosinophilia and gene rearrangements: Diagnostic pearls and pitfalls. Clinical Lymphoma, Myeloma & Leukemia. 2022;**22**:643-651

[33] Pozdnyakova O, Orazi A, Kelemen K, et al. Myeloid/lymphoid neoplasms associated with eosinophilia and rearrangements of PDGFRA, PDGFRB, or FGFR1 or with PCM1-JAK2.

American Journal of Clinical Pathology. 2021;**155**:160-178

[34] Khoury JD, Solary E, Abla O, et al. The 5th edition of the World Health Organization classification of haematolymphoid tumours: Myeloid and histiocytic/dendritic neoplasms. Leukemia. 2022;**36**:1703-1719

[35] Saft L, Kvasnicka HM, Boudova L, et al. Myeloid/lymphoid neoplasms with eosinophilia and tyrosine kinase fusion genes: A workshop report with focus on novel entities and a literature review including paediatric cases. Histopathology. 2023;**83**:829-849

[36] Arber DA, Orazi A, Hasserjian RP, et al. International consensus classification of myeloid neoplasms and acute leukemias: Integrating morphologic, clinical, and genomic data. Blood. 2022;**140**:1200-1228

[37] Kaur P, Khan WA. Chapter 8. Myeloid/lymphoid neoplasms with eosinophilia and platelet derived growth factor receptor alpha (PDGFRA) rearrangement. In: Leukemia [Internet]. Brisbane (AU): Exon Publications; 2022

[38] Rohmer J, Couteau-Chardon A, Trichereau J, et al. Epidemiology, clinical picture and long-term outcomes of FIP1L1-PDGFRA-positive myeloid neoplasm with eosinophilia: Data from 151 patients. American Journal of Hematology. 2020;**95**:1314-1323

[39] Helbig G. Myeloid/lymphoid neoplasms with eosinophilia: Clinical picture and therapeutic approaches. Acta Haematologica Polonica. 2021;**4**(52):272-277

[40] Jain N, Khoury JD, Pemmaraju N, et al. Imatinib therapy in a patient with suspected chronic neutrophilic leukemia and FIP1L1-PDGFRA rearrangement. Blood. 2013;**122**:3387-3388

[41] Akiely R, Almasri F, Almasri N, et al. A case report: Pediatric myeloid/lymphoid neoplasm with eosinophilia and PDGFRA rearrangement: The first case presenting as B-lymphoblastic lymphoma. Frontiers in Pediatrics. 2022;**10**:1059527

[42] Bellani V, Croci GA, Bucelli C, et al. Lymphomatoid papulosis associated with myeloid neoplasm with eosinophilia and FIP1L1::PDGFRA rearrangement: Successful imatinib treatment in two cases. The Journal of Dermatology. 2023;**50**:1330-1334

[43] Score J, Curtis C, Waghorn K, et al. Identification of a novel imatinib responsive KIF5B-PDGFRA fusion gene following screening for PDGFRA overexpression in patients with hypereosinophilia. Leukemia. 2006;**20**:827-832

[44] Walz C, Curtis C, Schnittger S, et al. Transient response to imatinib in a chronic eosinophilic leukemia associated with ins (9;4)(Q33;Q12q25) and a CDK5RAP2-PDGFRA fusion gene. Genes, Chromosomes & Cancer. 2006;**45**:950-956

[45] Curtis CE, Grand FH, Musto P, et al. Two novel imatinib-responsive PDGFRA fusion genes in chronic eosinophilic leukaemia. British Journal of Haematology. 2007;**138**:77-81

[46] Metzgeroth G, Steiner L, Naumann N, et al. Myeloid/lymphoid neoplasms with eosinophilia and tyrosine kinase gene fusions: Reevaluation of the defining characteristics in a registry-based cohort. Leukemia. 2023;**37**:1860-1867

[47] Jawhar M, Naumann N, Schwaab J, et al. Imatinib in myeloid/lymphoid neoplasms with eosinophilia and

rearrangement of PDGFRB in chronic or blast phase. Annals of Hematology. 2017;**96**:1463-1470

[48] Panagopoulos I, Brunetti M, Stoltenberg M, et al. Novel GTF2IPDGFRB and IKZF1-TYW1 fusions in pediatric leukemia with normal karyotype. Experimental Hematology & Oncology. 2019;**8**:12

[49] Jawhar M, Naumann N, Knut M, et al. Cytogenetically cryptic ZMYM2-FLT3 and DIAPH1-PDGFRB gene fusions in myeloid neoplasms with eosinophilia. Leukemia. 2017;**31**:2271-2273

[50] Kobayashi K, Mitsui K, Ichikawa H, et al. ATF7IP as a novel Pdgfrb fusion partner in acute lymphoblastic leukaemia in children. British Journal of Haematology. 2014;**165**:836-841

[51] Baer C, Muehlbacher V, Kern W, et al. Molecular genetic characterization of myeloid/lymphoid neoplasms associated with eosinophilia and rearrangement of PDGFRA, PDGFRB, FGFR1 or PCM1-JAK2. Haematologica. 2018;**103**:e348-e350

[52] Schwab C, Ryan SL, Chilton L, et al. EBF1-PDGFRB fusion in pediatric B-cell precursor acute lymphoblastic leukemia (BCP-ALL): Genetic profile and clinical İmplications. Blood. 2016;**127**:2214-2218

[53] Heilmann AM, Schrock AB, He J, et al. Novel PDGFRB fusions in childhood B-and T-acute lymphoblastic leukemia. Leukemia. 2017;**31**:1989-1992

[54] Maccaferri M, Pierini V, Di Giacomo D, et al. The importance of cytogenetic and molecular analyses in eosinophilia-associated myeloproliferative neoplasms: An unusual case with normal karyotype and TNIP1-PDGFRB rearrangement and overview of PDGFRB partner genes. Leukemia & Lymphoma. 2017;**58**:489-493

[55] Macdonald D, Reiter A, Cross NC. The 8p11 myeloproliferative syndrome: A distinct clinical entity caused by constitutive activation of FGFR1. Acta Haematologica. 2002;**107**:101-107

[56] Patnaik MM, Gangat N, Knudson RA, et al. Chromosome 8p11.2 translocations: Prevalence, fish analysis for FGFR1 and MYST3, and clinicopathologic correlates in a consecutive cohort of 13 cases from a single institution. American Journal of Hematology. 2010;**85**:238-242

[57] Tzankov A, Reichard KK, Hasserjian RP, et al. Updates on eosinophilic disorders. Virchows Archiv. 2023;**482**:85-97

[58] Jackson CC, Medeiros LJ, Miranda RN. 8p11 myeloproliferative syndrome: A review. Human Pathology. 2010;**41**:461-476

[59] Kumar KR, Chen W, Koduru PR, et al. Myeloid and lymphoid neoplasm with abnormalities of FGFR1 presenting with trilineage blasts and RUNX1 rearrangement: A case report and review of literature. American Journal of Clinical Pathology. 2015;**143**:738-748

[60] Strati P, Tang G, Duose DY, et al. Myeloid/lymphoid neoplasms with FGFR1 rearrangement. Leukemia & Lymphoma. 2018;**59**:1672-1676

[61] Yan Y, Qu S, Liu J, et al. Olverembatinib for myeloid/lymphoid neoplasm associated with eosinophilia and FGFR1 rearrangement. Leukemia & Lymphoma. 2023;**64**:1605-1610

[62] Ren M, Qin H, Ren R, et al. Ponatinib suppresses the development of myeloid

and lymphoid malignancies associated with FGFR1 abnormalities. Leukemia. 2013;**27**:32-40

[63] Chen J, DeAngelo DJ, Kutok JL, et al. PKC412 inhibits the zinc finger 198-fibroblast growth factor receptor 1 fusion tyrosine kinase and is active in treatment of stem cell myeloproliferative disorder. Proceedings of the National Academy of Sciences of the United States of America. 2004;**101**:14479-14484

[64] Kasbekar M, Nardi V, Cin D, et al. Targeted FGFR inhibition results in a durable remission in an FGFR1-driven myeloid neoplasm with eosinophilia. Blood Advances. 2020;**4**:3136-3140

[65] Stewart K, Carstairs KC, Dube ID, et al. Neutrophilic myelofibrosis presenting as Philadelphia chromosome negative Bcr non-rearranged chronic myeloid leukemia. American Journal of Hematology. 1990;**34**:59-63

[66] Roberts KG, Li Y, Payne-Turner D, et al. Targetable kinaseactivating lesions in Ph-like acute lymphoblastic leukemia. The New England Journal of Medicine. 2014;**371**:1005-1015

[67] Poitras JL, Dal Cin P, Aster JC, et al. Novel SSBP2-JAK2 fusion gene resulting from a T(5;9)(Q14.1;P24.1) in pre-B acute lymphocytic leukemia. Genes, Chromosomes & Cancer. 2008;**47**:884-889

[68] Tirado CA, Chen W, Huang LJ, et al. Novel JAK2 rearrangement resulting from a T(9;22) (P24;Q11.2) in B-acute lymphoblastic leukemia. Leukemia Research. 2010;**34**:1674-1676

[69] Luedke C, Rein L. Transformation to erythroblastic sarcoma from myeloid neoplasm with PCM1-JAK2. Blood. 2020;**136**:1113

[70] Snider JS, Znoyko I, Lindsey KG, et al. Integrated genomic analysis using chromosomal microarray, fluorescence in situ hybridization and mate pair analyses: Characterization of a cryptic T(9;22)(P24.1;Q11.2)/BCR-JAK2 in myeloid/lymphoid neoplasm with eosinophilia. Cancer Genetics. 2020:246-247; 44-47

[71] Chen JA, Hou Y, Roskin KM, et al. Lymphoid blast transformation in an Mpn with BCR-JAK2 treated with ruxolitinib: Putative mechanisms of resistance. Blood Advances. 2021;**5**:3492-3496

[72] Bain BJ, Ahmad S. Should myeloid and lymphoid neoplasms with PCM1-JAK2 and other rearrangements of JAK2 be recognized as specific entities? British Journal of Haematology. 2014;**166**:809-817

[73] Tang G, Sydney Sir Philip JK, Weinberg O, et al. Hematopoietic neoplasms with 9p24/JAK2 rearrangement: A multicenter study. Modern Pathology. 2019;**32**:490-498

[74] Rumi E, Milosevic JD, Casetti I, et al. Efficacy of ruxolitinib in chronic eosinophilic leukemia associated with a PCM1-JAK2 fusion gene. Journal of Clinical Oncology. 2013;**31**:e269-e271

[75] Lierman E, Selleslag D, Smits S, et al. Ruxolitinib inhibits transforming JAK2 fusion proteins *in vitro* and induces complete cytogenetic remission in t(8;9)(p22;p24)/PCM1-JAK2-positive chronic eosinophilic leukemia. Blood. 2012;**120**:1529-1531

[76] Reiter A, Walz C, Watmore A, et al. The T(8;9)(P22;P24) is a recurrent abnormality in chronic and acute leukemia that fuses PCM1 to JAK2. Cancer Research. 2005;**65**:2662-2667

[77] Peeters P, Raynaud SD, Cools J, et al. Fusion of TEL, the ETS variant gene 6 (ETV6), to the receptor-associated kinase JAK2 as a result of T(9;12) in a lymphoid and T(9;15;12) in a myeloid leukemia. Blood. 1997;**90**:2535-2540

[78] Schwaab J, Knut M, Haferlach C, et al. Limited duration of complete remission on ruxolitinib in myeloid neoplasms with PCM1-JAK2 and BCR-JAK2 fusion genes. Annals of Hematology. 2015;**94**:233-238

[79] Tang G, Tam W, Short NJ, et al. Myeloid/lymphoid neoplasms with FLT3 rearrangement. Modern Pathology. 2021;**34**:1673-1685

[80] Schoelinck J, Gervasoni J, Guillermin Y, et al. T cell phenotype and lack of eosinophilia are not uncommon in extramedullary myeloid/lymphoid neoplasms with ETV6::FLT3 fusion: A case report and review of the literature. Virchows Archiv. 2024;**484**(5):853-857

[81] Yao J, Xu L, Aypar U, et al. Myeloid/lymphoid neoplasms with eosinophilia/basophilia and ETV6-ABL1 fusion: cell-of-origin and response to tyrosine kinase inhibition. Haematologica. 2021;**106**:614-618

[82] Xie W, Wang SA, Hu S, et al. Myeloproliferative neoplasm with ABL1/ETV6 rearrangement mimics chronic myeloid leukemia and responds to tyrosine kinase inhibitors. Cancer Genetics. 2018;**228-229**:41-46

[83] Yamamoto K, Yakushijin K, Nakamachi Y, et al. Extramedullary T-lymphoid blast crisis of an ETV6/ABL1-positive myeloproliferative neoplasm with T(9;12)(Q34;P13) and T(7;14) (P13;Q11.2). Annals of Hematology. 2014;**93**:1435-1438

[84] Gancheva K, Virchis A, Howard-Reeves J, et al. Myeloproliferative neoplasm with ETV6-ABL1 fusion: A case report and literatüre review. Molecular Cytogenetics. 2013;**6**:39

[85] Cessna MH, Paulraj P, Hilton B, et al. Chronic myelomonocytic leukemia with ETV6-ABL1 rearrangement and SMC1A mutation. Cancer Genetics. 2019;**238**:31-36

[86] Zaliova M, Moorman AV, Cazzaniga G, et al. Characterization of leukemias with ETV6-ABL1 fusion. Haematologica. 2016;**101**:1082-1093

[87] Sangle NA, Perkins SL. Core-binding factor acute myeloid leukemia. Archives of Pathology & Laboratory Medicine. 2011;**135**:1504-1509

[88] Yin CC, Medeiros LJ, Bueso-Ramos CE. Recent advances in the diagnosis and classification of myeloid neoplasms—comments on the 2008 WHO classification. International Journal of Laboratory Hematology. 2010;**32**(5):461-476

[89] Arber D, Vardiman J, Brunning R, et al. Acute myeloid leukemia with recurrent genetic abnormalities. In: Swerlow SH, Campo E, Harris NL, et al., editors. WHO Classification of Tumours of Haematopoietic and Lymphoid Tissues. Lyon, France: IARC Press; 2008. pp. 110-123. World Health Organization Classification of Tumours; Vol 2

[90] Marcucci G, Mrozek K, Ruppert AS, et al. Prognostic factors and outcome of core binding factor acute myeloid leukemia patients with T(8;21) differ from those of patients with Inv(16): A cancer and leukemia group B study. Journal of Clinical Oncology. 2005;**23**(24):5705-5717

[91] Appelbaum FR, Kopecky KJ, Tallman MS, et al. The clinical spectrum of adult acute myeloid leukaemia associated with core binding factor translocations. British Journal of Haematology. 2006;**135**(2):165-173

[92] Naymagon L, Marcellino B, Mascarenhas J. Eosinophilia in acute myeloid leukemia: Overlooked and underexamined. Blood Reviews. 2019;**36**:23-31

[93] Larson RA, Williams SF, Le Beau MM, et al. Acute myelomonocytic leukemia with abnormal eosinophils and Inv(16) or t(16;16) has a favorable prognosis. Blood. 1986;**68**:1242-1249

[94] Swirsky DM, Li YS, Matthews JG, et al. 8;21 translocation in acute granulocytic leukaemia: Cytological, cytochemical and clinical features. British Journal of Haematology. 1984;**56**:199-213

[95] Haferlach T, Bennett JM, Loffler H, et al. Acute myeloid leukemia with translocation (8;21). Cytomorphology, dysplasia, and prognostic factors in 41 cases. AML cooperative group and ECOG. Leukemia & Lymphoma. 1996;**23**:227-234

[96] Merchant SH, Haines S, Hall B, et al. Fluorescence in situ hybridization identifies cryptic T(16;16)(P13;Q22) masked by Del(16)(Q22) in a case of AML-M4 Eo. The Journal of Molecular Diagnostics. 2004;**6**(3):271-274

[97] Paschka P, Marcucci G, Ruppert AS, et al. Adverse prognostic significance of KIT mutations in adult acute myeloid leukemia with inv(16) and t(8;21): A cancer and leukemia group B study. Journal of Clinical Oncology. 2006;**24**(24):3904-3911

[98] Marcucci G. Core binding factor acute myeloid leukemia. Clinical Advances in Hematology & Oncology. 2006;**4**(5):339-341

[99] Schoch C, Haase D, Haferlach T, et al. Fifty-one patients with acute myeloid leukemia and translocation t(8;21)(q22;q22): An additional deletion in 9q is an adverse prognostic factor. Leukemia. 1996;**10**(8):1288-1295

[100] Brockow K. Epidemiology, prognosis, and risk factors in mastocytosis. Immunology and Allergy Clinics of North America. 2014;**34**:283

[101] Méni C, Bruneau J, Georgin-Lavialle S, et al. Paediatric mastocytosis: A systematic review of 1747 cases. The British Journal of Dermatology. 2015;**172**:642

[102] Wolff K, Komar M, Petzelbauer P. Clinical and histopathological aspects of cutaneous mastocytosis. Leukemia Research. 2001;**25**:519

[103] Cruse G, Metcalfe DD, Olivera A. Functional deregulation of KIT: Link to mast cell proliferative diseases and other neoplasms. Immunology and Allergy Clinics of North America. 2014;**34**:219

[104] Bibi S, Langenfeld F, Jeanningros S, at al. Molecular defects in mastocytosis: KIT and beyond KIT. Immunology and Allergy Clinics of North America. 2014;**34**:239

[105] Longley BJ Jr, Morganroth GS, Tyrrell L, et al. Altered metabolism of mast-cell growth factor (C-kit ligand) in cutaneous mastocytosis. The New England Journal of Medicine. 1993;**328**:1302

[106] Castells MC, Hornick JL, Akin C. Anaphylaxis after hymenoptera sting: Is it venom allergy, a clonal disorder, or both? The Journal of Allergy and Clinical Immunology. In Practice. 2015;**3**:350

[107] Bonadonna P, Bonifacio M, Lombardo C, et al. Hymenoptera anaphylaxis and C-kit mutations: An unexpected association. Current Allergy and Asthma Reports. 2015;**15**:49

[108] Zanotti R, Lombardo C, Passalacqua G, et al. Clonal mast cell disorders in patients with severe hymenoptera venom allergy and normal serum tryptase levels. The Journal of Allergy and Clinical Immunology. 2015;**136**:135

[109] Alvarez-Twose I, Zanotti R, González-De-Olano D, et al. Nonaggressive systemic mastocytosis (SM) without skin lesions associated with insect-induced anaphylaxis shows unique features versus other indolent SM. The Journal of Allergy and Clinical Immunology. 2014;**133**:520

[110] Rossini M, Zanotti R, Viapiana O, et al. Bone involvement and osteoporosis in mastocytosis. Immunology and Allergy Clinics of North America. 2014;**34**:383

[111] King JJ, Crawford EA, Iwenofu OH, Fox EJ. Case report: Pathologic long bone fracture in a patient with systemic mastocytosis. Clinical Orthopaedics and Related Research. 2007;**459**:263

[112] Lim KH, Tefferi A, Lasho TL, et al. Systemic mastocytosis In 342 consecutive adults: Survival studies and prognostic factors. Blood. 2009;**113**:5727

[113] Pardanani A. Systemic mastocytosis in adults: 2015 update on diagnosis, risk stratification, and management. American Journal of Hematology. 2015;**90**:250

[114] Wimmer J, Hurstel R. Systemic mastocytosis with an associated T(8;21) (Q22;Q22) acute myeloid leukemia. Blood. 2021;**137**:2564

[115] Parker RI. Hematologic aspects of systemic mastocytosis. Hematology/Oncology Clinics of North America. 2000;**14**:557

[116] Maric I, Robyn J, Metcalfe DD, et al. KIT D816V-associated systemic mastocytosis with eosinophilia and FIP1L1/PDGFRA-associated chronic eosinophilic leukemia are distinct entities. The Journal of Allergy and Clinical Immunology. 2007;**120**(3):680-687

[117] Pardanani A, Lim KH, Lasho TL, et al. Prognostically relevant breakdown of 123 patients with systemic mastocytosis associated with other myeloid malignancies. Blood. 2009;**114**(18):3769-3772

[118] Akin C, Kirshenbaum AS, Semere T, et al. Analysis of the surface expression of C-kit and occurrence of the C-kit Asp816Val activating mutation in T cells, B cells, and myelomonocytic cells in patients with mastocytosis. Experimental Hematology. 2000;**28**(2):140-147

[119] Yavuz AS, Lipsky PE, Yavuz S, et al. Evidence for the involvement of a hematopoietic progenitor cell in systemic mastocytosis from single-cell analysis of mutations in the C-kit gene. Blood. 2002;**100**(2):661-665

[120] Leguit RJ, Wang SA, George TI, et al. The international consensus classification of mastocytosis and related entities. Virchows Archiv. 2023;**482**:99-112

[121] Morgado JM, Perbellini O, Johnson RC, et al. CD30 expression by bone marrow mast cells from different diagnostic variants of systemic mastocytosis. Histopathology. 2013;**63**:780-787

[122] Gotlib V, Darji J, Bloomfield K, et al. Eosinophilic variant of chronic

myeloid leukemia with vascular complications. Leukemia & Lymphoma. 2003;**44**(9):1609-1613

[123] Faldu P, Yousuf M, Abdelmagid M, et al. Basophilia and eosinophilia in polycythemia vera and essential thrombocythemia: Clinical, genotype, and prognostic correlates. Annals of Hematology. 2025;**104**(6):3223-3234

[124] Kumar A, Sinha S, Tripathi AK. Chronic eosinophilic leukemia: A case report and review of literature. Indian Journal of Hematology and Blood Transfusion. 2007;**23**(3-4):112-115

[125] Morsia E, Reichard K, Pardanani A, et al. WHO defined chronic eosinophilic leukemia, not otherwise specified (CEL, NOS): A contemporary series from the Mayo Clinic. American Journal of Hematology. 2020;**95**:E172-E174

[126] Onida F, Chalandon Y, Carreras E, et al. Chapter 75. Myelodysplastic/myeloproliferative neoplasms. In: The EBMT Handbook: Hematopoietic Stem Cell Transplantation and Cellular Therapies [Internet]. 7th ed. Cham (CH): Springer; 2019

[127] Jin JJ, Butterfield JH, Weiler CR. Hematologic malignancies identified in patients with hypereosinophilia and hypereosinophilic syndromes. The Journal of Allergy and Clinical Immunology. In Practice. 2015;**3**:920

[128] Greer JP, York JC, Cousar JB, et al. Peripheral T-cell lymphoma: A clinicopathologic study of 42 cases. Journal of Clinical Oncology. 1984;**2**:788

[129] Roufosse F, Garaud S, de Leval L. Lymphoproliferative disorders associated with hypereosinophilia. Seminars in Hematology. 2012;**49**:138-148

[130] Tancrède-Bohin E, Ionescu MA, de La Salmonière P, et al. Prognostic value of blood eosinophilia in primary cutaneous T-cell lymphomas. Archives of Dermatology. 2004;**140**:1057-1061

[131] Robyn J, Noel P, Wlodarska I, et al. Imatinib-responsive hypereosinophilia in a patient with B cell ALL. Leukemia & Lymphoma. 2004;**45**:2497

[132] Toboso DG, Campos CB. Peripheral eosinophilia as the first manifestation of B-cell acute lymphoblastic leukemia with t(5;14)(q31;q32). Blood. 2017;**130**:380

[133] Lefèvre G, Copin MC, Staumont-Sallé D, et al. The lymphoid variant of hypereosinophilic syndrome: Study of 21 patients with CD3-CD4+ aberrant T-cell phenotype. Medicine (Baltimore). 2014;**93**:255

[134] Simon HU, Plötz SG, Dummer R, Blaser K. Abnormal clones of T cells producing interleukin-5 in idiopathic eosinophilia. The New England Journal of Medicine. 1999;**341**:1112

Chapter 5

Eosinophils and Basophils in Breast Cancer, the Neglected Players?

Claudia A. Garay-Canales, Raul Aragon-Franco, Yair Rodríguez-Santiago, Diana L. Ruiz-Antonio, María del Sol Ríos-Avila, César A. Zavala-López, Karen E. Nava-Castro and Jorge Morales-Montor

Abstract

Breast cancer (BC) is the most common cancer and the leading cause of cancer-related mortality among women globally. This heterogeneous group of diseases can be clinically classified into three subtypes: luminal, HER-2, and triple-negative breast cancers (TNBCs). The immune system plays a pivotal role in the development and progression of cancer, with eosinophils and basophils being under-estimated players. Although constituting less than 1–5% of circulating leukocytes, these cells can directly act on cancer cells through cell surface receptors, releasing cytotoxic granule proteins and producing immunoregulatory mediators. Recent studies have shown that circulating eosinophilia and tumor tissue infiltration by eosinophils are associated with a favorable prognostic factor, particularly in patients undergoing concomitant therapy for HER-2-positive and TNBC. Immunotherapy, including neoadjuvant chemotherapy and immune checkpoint blockade, has demonstrated that elevated circulating eosinophils and tumor-associated tissue eosinophilia (TATE) are predictive of a more favorable treatment response. Although the study of basophils has been limited due to their rarity, emerging evidence suggests they play a role in various cancers, with ongoing investigations exploring their involvement in breast cancer. A more comprehensive understanding of the roles of eosinophils and basophils in breast cancer may facilitate the development of targeted therapies. The presence or absence of these cells within the tumor environment could indicate the efficacy or failure of some new treatments for breast cancer. Further research is necessary to elucidate the mechanisms underlying the interplay between these immune cells and breast cancer.

Keywords: breast cancer, eosinophils, basophils, TATE, prognosis, biomarker, immune checkpoint blockade

1. Introduction

Breast cancer (BC) is the most common cancer and the leading cause of cancer-related mortality among women globally, with incidence rates increasing annually in many countries over recent decades [1]. This cancer develops from the uncontrolled growth of cells and their ability to evade antitumor defenses, leading to tumor formation in different breast portions, including lobules, ducts, and connective tissue. In 2022 alone, BC was responsible for about 2.3 million new cases and 670,000 deaths worldwide, highlighting its status as the most common and widespread cancer among women [2]. The established risk factors include genetic predisposition (such as BRCA mutations), environmental pollutant exposure, family history, aging, ethnicity, higher body mass index (BMI), and nulliparity [3].

BC predominantly affects women, but it also occurs in men, albeit rarely, accounting for approximately 1% of all breast cancer cases. Despite its low incidence, male breast cancer has been increasing in recent years. Moreover, men with BC tend to have poorer outcomes, often being diagnosed at a more advanced stage, with fewer treatment options and a worse overall prognosis compared to women [4, 5].

1.1 Classification (subtypes)

BC arises from the uncontrolled proliferation of a group of cells in different regions of the breast, known as adenocarcinomas. These cancer cells can be confined to the breast tissue (in situ) or can become invasive, spreading to surrounding tissues or metastasizing to distant peripheral tissues. The most common types are ductal carcinoma, which develops at the edge of the duct that carries milk from the lobules of the breast to the nipple, and lobular carcinoma, which develops in the lobules. Breast tumors are categorized by histology and immunohistochemistry, based on American Society of Clinical Oncology (ASCO) guidelines, which include estrogen receptor (ER), progesterone receptor (PR), human epidermal growth factor receptor 2 (HER-2), and triple-negative breast cancer (TNBC). Gene expression profiling of breast carcinoma also allows for primary classification in at least four distinct "intrinsic" subtypes, including two ER-positive (luminal A and luminal B) and two ER-negative (ERBB-2 and basal subtypes) groups [6]. TNBC is defined by the absence of hormone receptors (ER < 1% and PR < 20%) and HER-2 (≤10%) and represents 10% of all BC cases. TNBC is the most aggressive among the four subtypes of BC, with the highest proliferation indicated by an index of Ki-67 protein >30% present only in dividing cells and a poorer prognosis, and it is usually related to invasive ductal carcinoma and variants of apocrine and metaplastic carcinomas. Several studies of gene expression revealed that TNBC is highly heterogeneous and can be divided into seven different subtypes [7].

This disease exhibits multiple etiologies that require further studies to understand its molecular and cellular underpinnings and risk factors [8]. The immune system is dedicated to recognizing tumor cells and triggering diverse mechanisms to eradicate them (immunosurveillance). Cytotoxic T lymphocytes (CTLs) recognize and eliminate tumor cells through cell-to-cell interactions, targeting cells presenting foreign major histocompatibility complex class I (MHC-I) molecules. However, some tumor cells evade CTL recognition by downregulating MHC-I expression. Conversely, natural killer (NK) cells recognize and target cells with low MHC-I expression, thereby complementing CTL-mediated immunity. As a result, NK cells and CTLs play critical roles in antitumor immunity [9]. Despite the crucial role of these immune cells, cancer cells have developed diverse mechanisms to evade immune recognition and response, underscoring the need to study the involvement of additional immune cells, such as eosinophils and basophils, which possess potent cytotoxic capabilities.

In healthy individuals, eosinophils are present in relatively low numbers, typically accounting for less than 5% of peripheral white blood cells, and exhibit a restricted lifespan of 8–18 hours in circulation and 3–4 days in tissues. They primarily reside in tissues including the gastrointestinal tract, lung parenchyma, mammary gland lobules, and uterine endometrium. While their roles in innate and adaptive immunity against helminth infections, asthma, and allergic disorders are well-defined, their role against specific pathogens and cancer remains incompletely characterized. Critically, emerging evidence underscores their involvement in cancer progression, where they exhibit context-dependent roles in tumor progression, immune modulation, and therapeutic responses [10–12].

Basophils are a rare subset of white blood cells, comprising 1% or less of circulating leukocytes, with a relatively short lifespan of approximately 60 hours. They are distributed in the lungs, skin, kidneys, and heart. Owing to their morphological and functional similarities with tissue-resident mast cells, basophils were initially misclassified as their circulating precursors or counterparts of mast cells. This misconception, combined with their scarcity, has hindered the study of basophils, resulting in a limited understanding of their role in diverse inflammatory and infectious diseases, as well as cancer, which remains to be further elucidated [13–16].

2. Does the tumor microenvironment include eosinophils and basophils?

The tumor microenvironment (TME) is a complex milieu comprising extracellular matrix components, stromal cells, and infiltrated cells from the immune system, including tumor-associated macrophages (TAMs), tumor-infiltrated neutrophils (TANs), mast cells, NKs, and tumor-infiltrating lymphocytes [17, 18]. The breast tumor microenvironment has been extensively reviewed elsewhere [18–22]. TME is a key factor in tumor growth, progression, and resistance to therapy. Identifying TME components and understanding how they interact has enabled the identification of prognostic biomarkers, potential therapeutic targets, and effective treatment strategies [23].

In BC, the tumor shows high levels of leukocyte infiltration [24]. It can both suppress or promote tumor progression, depending on the cancer subtype and the balance between immune cell types and their functional state (active or suppressive) [25]. In general, lymphocytes $CD4^+$ T helper 1 and $CD8^+$ T cytotoxic, NK cells, M1 macrophages, and dendritic cells (DCs) have antitumoral effects; meanwhile, T helper lymphocytes $FOXP3^+$, $CD4^+$ Th2 cells, M2 macrophages, and myeloid-derived suppressor cells (MDSCs) are pro-tumoral [26]. Tumor-infiltrating lymphocytes are a prognostic marker for pathological complete responses (pCRs) in all BC subtypes [27] as well as for better survival in TNBC and HER-2^+ subtypes [26]. Only in luminal subtypes is the higher ratio of $FOXP3^+/CD8^+$ predictive of a worse prognosis [28].

The TME immune cell pattern varies significantly from individual to individual and by molecular subtype [29]. TNBC and HER-2 tend to have higher tumor-infiltrating lymphocytes [29, 30], while luminal tumors tend to have lower infiltration but higher levels of immunosuppressive cells. Among that infiltration, there is high expression of $FOXP3^+$ (Treg cells), $CD68^+$, $CD163^+$ TAMs, $CD4^+$, and $CD8^+$ [30, 31]. In ER- tumors, there is a higher percentage of M2 macrophages and $CD163^+$ TAMs [31]. Other immune cells found in the TME of BC are Tγδ cells, T follicular cells (Tfh), Th17 cells, B lymphocytes, TANs, NKs, DCs, MDSC, and innate lymphoid cells (ILCs) [31].

The role of eosinophils and basophils in human BC remained in the dark, first because they were found to be very low in the TME. However, a slight increase was observed after neoadjuvant chemotherapy administration, especially in FcεR1α$^+$/CD117−/CD11b−/CD49d$^+$ basophils [24]. Similarly, immune checkpoint blockade (ICB) treatment increased myelopoiesis and systemic eosinophil production. Moreover, IL-33 is induced after ICB + cisplatin, eosinophils are recruited to the TME, and the expression of the SINGLEC8 marker and eosinophil-related genes increased intratumorally in responders but not in non-responders' mice. This is correlated with increased expression of CD8$^+$ T cell-related genes, suggesting a favorable synergistic response to treatment [32]. Then, eosinophils and basophils could play a key role during the progression or treatment response to tumors.

3. Eosinophils

Eosinophils are granulocytic leukocytes originally described by Paul Ehrlich, characterized by cytoplasmic granules that stain with eosin and a multilobed nucleus [33–35]. These cells express several surface markers, including CD49D, CD61, and CCR3, while activated eosinophils increase the expression of adhesion and signaling molecules such as CD11b, CD18, and CD69 [11]. Their persistence in tissues is regulated by cytokines, including IL-3, IL-5, IL-9, IL-13, IL-15, and GM-CSF, which inhibit apoptosis and prolong their survival [11, 12, 36].

Eosinophils contain granules rich in cytotoxic proteins—such as major basic protein (MBP), eosinophil cationic protein (ECP), eosinophil peroxidase (EPO), and eosinophil-derived neurotoxin (EDN)—and can rapidly release cytokines, inflammatory mediators, and eosinophil extracellular traps (EETs), contributing to host defense and immune regulation [11, 33, 37]. In addition, eosinophil responses can be modulated by sex hormones such as estradiol and testosterone, modulating biological processes such as chemotaxis, apoptosis, degranulation, and adhesion [36, 38–40].

Eosinophils and macrophages are essential for mammary gland development in mice. Gouon-Evans et al. observed that these cells localized to the terminal end bud (TEB), with macrophages concentrated at the neck and eosinophils at the distal end. Using CFS1-deficient and CCL11-deficient mouse models, they showed that macrophages are crucial for TEB elongation, while eosinophils are necessary for TEB branching. Notably, eosinophil depletion did not affect macrophage populations, and conversely, eosinophil overproduction (*via* IL-5 overexpression) resulted in transiently impaired branching morphogenesis. Estrogen and progesterone were found to contribute to the recruitment of these immune cells to the developing mammary gland [41].

3.1 Eosinophils in cancer

The response of eosinophils to cancer cells is multifaceted. As illustrated in **Figure 1**, eosinophils exhibit dual and opposing roles within the TME, exerting both antitumoral and pro-tumoral effects in a context-dependent manner. The function of eosinophils in cancer is intricately linked to the specific characteristics of the TME. At the early stage of tumor formation, eosinophils can infiltrate tumors upon activation of the IL-5Rα/CCR3 pathway and in response to chemokines such as eotaxins

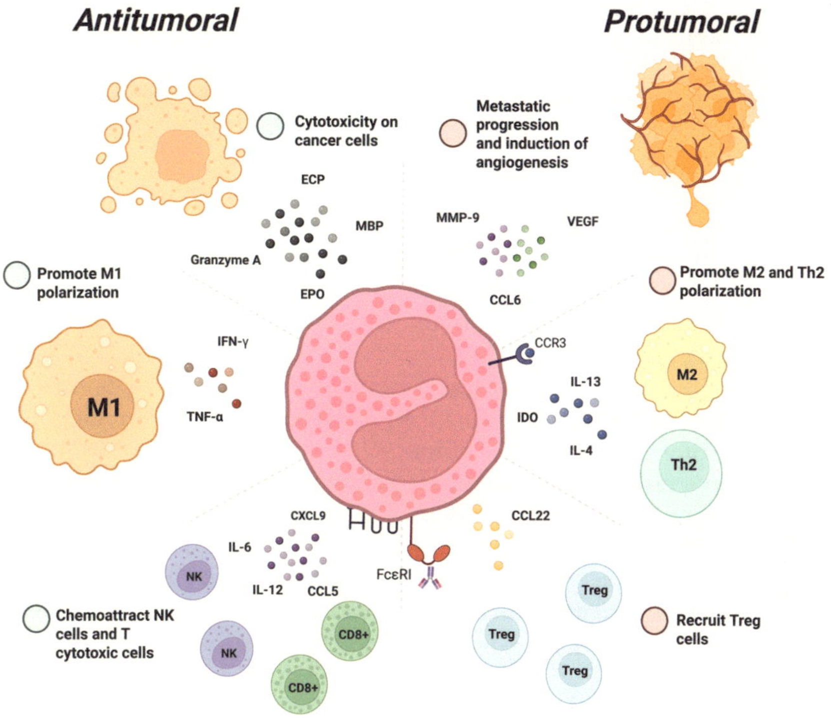

Figure 1.
Dual role of eosinophils in cancer: Antitumoral or pro-tumoral activity. The antitumor activity is performed by the release of cytotoxic granule proteins or indirectly by modulating immune responses, including the recruitment of CD8⁺ T cells, NK cells, the maturation of dendritic cells, and the polarization of macrophages to an M1 phenotype. The pro-tumoral functions are exerted through the secretion of TGF-β1, IL-6, IL-8, VEGF, and MMP-9. Eosinophils can promote angiogenesis, tissue remodeling, fibroblast proliferation, and the formation of metastatic niches. Created in https://BioRender.com.

(CCL11, CCL24, and CCL26) produced by tumor cells, leading to their accumulation in various cancers, including lung, colorectal, and melanoma [10].

The antitumor activity of eosinophils is achieved through the release of cytotoxic granule proteins or indirectly by modulating immune responses, including the recruitment of $CD8^+$ T cells, NK cells, the maturation of dendritic cells, and the polarization of macrophages to an M1 phenotype. Afterward, if the immune response is unable to eliminate all cancer cells, the tumor can proliferate, and the role of eosinophils shifts to a pro-tumoral phenotype. These eosinophils exert the pro-tumoral functions through the secretion of factors such as TGF-β1, IL-6, IL-8, VEGF, and MMP-9. Eosinophils can promote angiogenesis, tissue remodeling, fibroblast proliferation, and the formation of metastatic niches, which favor tumor development [42].

On the other hand, clinically, elevated eosinophil counts have been associated with improved prognosis in several cancers, including bladder, colorectal, prostate, breast, and oral squamous-cell carcinoma. In contrast, in cancers such as melanoma and non-small-cell lung cancer, eosinophilia may correlate with tumor progression by promoting M2 macrophage polarization, recruitment of regulatory T cells, and Th2 differentiation [10, 11, 43–45].

3.2 Eosinophils in breast cancer

The infiltration of eosinophils into tumor tissue is known as tumor-associated tissue eosinophilia (TATE), a phenomenon first described in the late nineteenth century and generally associated with a favorable prognosis in several carcinomas [46]. In BC, immunohistochemical analyses have detected deposits of eosinophil peroxidase (EPO) in approximately 88% of tumor samples, indicating intense eosinophil activity within the TME [47]. As depicted in **Figure 2**, eosinophils can act by promoting pro-tumoral and antitumoral responses: on the pro-tumoral side, through VEGF-A-driven angiogenesis, IL-4-mediated M2 polarization, and MMP9-facilitated metastasis; on the antitumoral side, eosinophils act through the release of cytotoxic proteins, cytokines, and histamine, the recruitment of $CD8^{+}$ T cells, and the formation of eosinophil extracellular traps (EETs).

In addition, biopsies of ductal breast carcinoma have revealed abundant eosinophils adjacent to the tumor, suggesting their involvement in the local immune response [48]. Interestingly, in BC, eosinophil infiltration is predominantly found within the tumor rather than in the surrounding stroma, and its prevalence may vary depending on the molecular subtype. For example, stromal eosinophils appear less frequently in tumors with high estrogen receptor expression, whereas no clear association has been observed with progesterone receptor or HER-2 status [49]. The presence of intratumoral or stromal eosinophils correlates positively with tumor stage and primary tumor size.

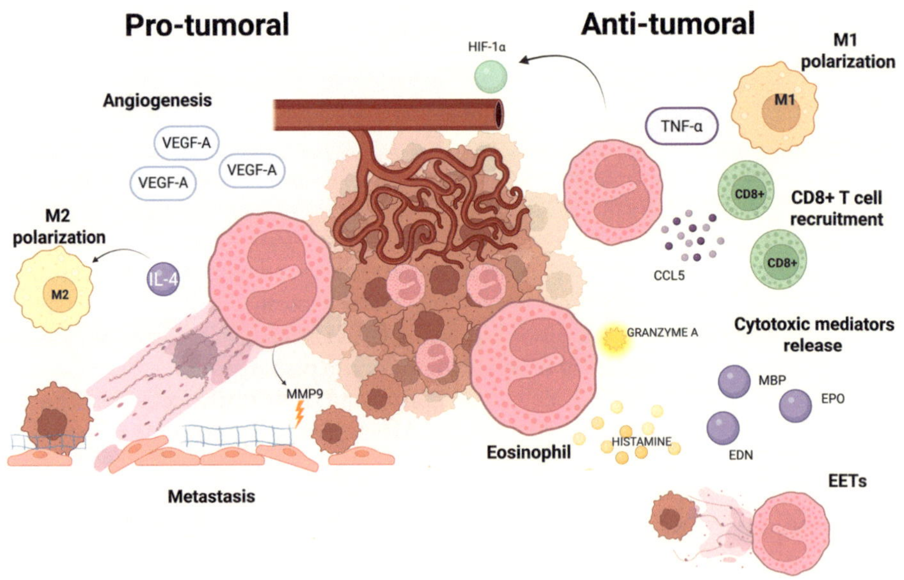

Figure 2.
Eosinophils exhibit dual roles in breast cancer, promoting both pro-tumoral and antitumoral responses. On the pro-tumoral side, eosinophils act through VEGF-A-driven angiogenesis, IL-4-mediated M2 polarization, and MMP9-facilitated metastasis; on the antitumoral side, eosinophils act through the release of cytotoxic proteins, cytokines, and histamine, the recruitment of $CD8^{+}$ T cells, and the formation of eosinophil extracellular traps (EETs) through cytokine/chemokine degranulation and the formation of eosinophil extracellular traps (EETs). Created in https://BioRender.com.

Usually, eosinophils are scarce, making it difficult to detect them by routine hematoxylin–eosin staining of BC biopsies, which hinders the consistent assessment of their role in prognosis. To overcome this obstacle, transcriptomic analysis using the computational algorithm CIBERSORT revealed a better outcome when eosinophil infiltration was detected [50]. From the Cancer Genome Atlas (TCGA) dataset BC cohort, 3.7% of TATE was detected, with a different proportion depending on the BC subtype (32.5% luminal, 5% HER-2-positive, and 15% TNBC subtypes). In patients with TATE+, the TME exhibited distinct characteristics, including an increase in T helper cells and monocytes, accompanied by a decrease in mast cells, B cells, and resting $CD4^+$ T cells. Notably, this compositional shift was associated with improved disease-free survival; however, the results are not yet statistically significant [51].

Recent studies suggest that eosinophils may enhance the efficacy of antitumor therapies, particularly in the context of immunotherapy. In patients with TNBC treated with nivolumab, systemic accumulation of eosinophils was associated with improved progression-free and overall survival, as well as increased activation of $CD8^+$ T cells. This effect appears to be mediated by cytokines such as IL-5 and IL-33 produced by $CD4^+$ T cells, which promote eosinophil recruitment and activation within the TME [32].

Experimental depletion of eosinophils reduced $CD8^+$ T-cell activation and abolished the synergistic effect observed between chemotherapy and immunotherapy, highlighting their functional role in treatment response. Although the mechanisms underlying these effects remain incompletely understood, emerging evidence suggests that targeting eosinophil recruitment could represent a promising therapeutic strategy. For instance, the DPP4 (CD26) inhibitor sitagliptin has been shown to induce tumor-derived IL-33 release and promote eosinophil infiltration in several solid tumors, including BC models [52]. These findings support the potential development of eosinophil-based therapeutic approaches aimed at enhancing antitumor immune responses and improving treatment efficacy.

4. Basophils

Basophils in mice and humans are identified by the expression of CCR3, CD39b, IL-3R (CD123), CD45, FcεRIa, and their lack of tyrosine kinase receptor expression, which is a signature surface marker of mast cells [15, 53]. Basophil activation may occur *via* IgE antibodies and IL-3, or *via* pathogen-associated molecular patterns recognized by Toll-like receptors. Diverse chemokines, including RANTES, eotaxins, and MCPs mediate its migration. In inflammatory situations, activated basophils release the contents of their granules, predominantly histamine, which induces vascular permeability, smooth muscle contraction, as well as leukotrienes (LTC4) and interleukins [14, 15, 53–55], which, together, promote the polarization of type 2 response in T $CD4^+$ and $CD8^+$. Furthermore, they induce B cells to synthesize IgE through several effector molecules, including IL-4, IL-5, IL-6, IL-9, chemokines, basogranulin, and granzyme B.

The effect of sex hormones on basophils is barely described; estradiol alone induces the degranulation of preformed mediators; however, estradiol strongly potentiates the effects, as does the release of histamine in the presence of IgE. These estrogenic effects are mediated by ER-α activation [56, 57]. For many years, the role of this leukocyte has been focused on allergic responses and helminthic infections. More recently, they have been recognized for their immunoregulatory role in tumor growth, the metastasis of different types of cancer, and the anti- and pro-tumor immune responses.

4.1 Basophils in cancer

One of the most relevant functions of activated human basophils is their ability to release significant amounts of VEGF-A and VEGF-B [58]. Vascular endothelial growth factor (VEGF) is a key mediator for the stimulation of angiogenesis, and its upregulation in cancer has been associated with the development of tumor vessels, which, although irregular and disorganized [59], fulfill the function of providing nutrients for the proliferation and spread of tumor cells [60]. In particular, the VEGF-A is one of the most potent pro-angiogenic molecules due to its high tissue diffusion capacity and affinity for the main angiogenesis receptor, VEGFR-2, which together promote the branching and extension of blood vessels capable of supplying the tumor [61]. In certain types of solid cancers, this binding is significantly enhanced by the co-receptor Neuropilin-1 (NRP1), which increases the intensity and duration of the pro-angiogenic signal and contributes to the chemotaxis of endothelial cells toward VEGF gradients [62].

Basophils not only contribute to providing the tumor with the necessary means to obtain nutrients, but can also modulate the cytokine profile faced by cancer cells. When activated, basophils release IL-4, which interacts with the IL-4Rα receptor in naïve T cells and triggers the JAK-STAT6 signaling cascade, which, in turn, activates the GATA3 gene. This gene is closely related to the differentiation of cells toward Th2 profiles, in addition to inducing the production of more IL-4, which amplifies the Th2 response [63]. This new source of IL-4 secretion, under specific conditions, and the production of chemokines such as CCL3 and CCL4 can promote positive feedback that reinforces the presence of the Th2 profile by stimulating more immune system cells, including eosinophils, mast cells, M2 macrophages, and B lymphocytes. Together, this sustained process can promote the inhibition of cytotoxic immune responses against cancer cells [64–66].

Another mechanism by which basophils may contribute to the proliferation or inhibition of tumor cells is through the formation of extracellular DNA traps. Basophil Extracellular Traps (BETs) are mitochondrial and granulocytic DNA structures that can be activated by IgE or C5a [67] and, although these have been little studied, in general, extracellular traps have been associated with a complex series of mechanisms capable of promoting metastasis progression, angiogenesis, and immunomodulation [68–70], so it could be inferred that BETs could also be involved in cancer progression. On the other hand, these same pro-tumor factors may be associated with antitumor functions. In animal models of melanoma, the almost total depletion of regulatory T cells (Tregs) triggers a sharp increase in infiltrating basophils, which precedes the massive arrival of $CD8^+$ T lymphocytes in the tumor microenvironment. These basophils produce significant amounts of CCL3 and CCL4 chemokines, which are directly responsible for attracting $CD8^+$ cells, promoting cytotoxic lymphocyte-dependent tumor regression [71]. Clinical studies of ovarian cancer have shown that a higher proportion of circulating basophils is associated with better overall and progression-free survival rates [72].

These studies suggest that, under appropriate activation conditions, basophils act not only as direct effector cells but also as regulators of the microenvironment that drive effective cytotoxic responses. In addition, these granulocytes can release cytotoxic mediators such as granzyme B, TNF-α, and histamine, which can exert direct effects against tumor cells [73]. Additionally, the presence of IL-33 in the tumor microenvironment can activate basophils, leading to the increased expression of granzyme B and enhanced cytotoxic capacity, as evidenced by *in vitro* melanoma cell death. This functional capacity is highly dependent on the immunological context. As represented in **Figure 3**, basophils can shift between pro- and antitumoral roles through mechanisms that range from VEGF-driven angiogenesis and IgE-mediated degranulation to chemokine-directed immune infiltration and the release of extracellular traps. In a Th1-type inflammatory environment, basophils are recruited by

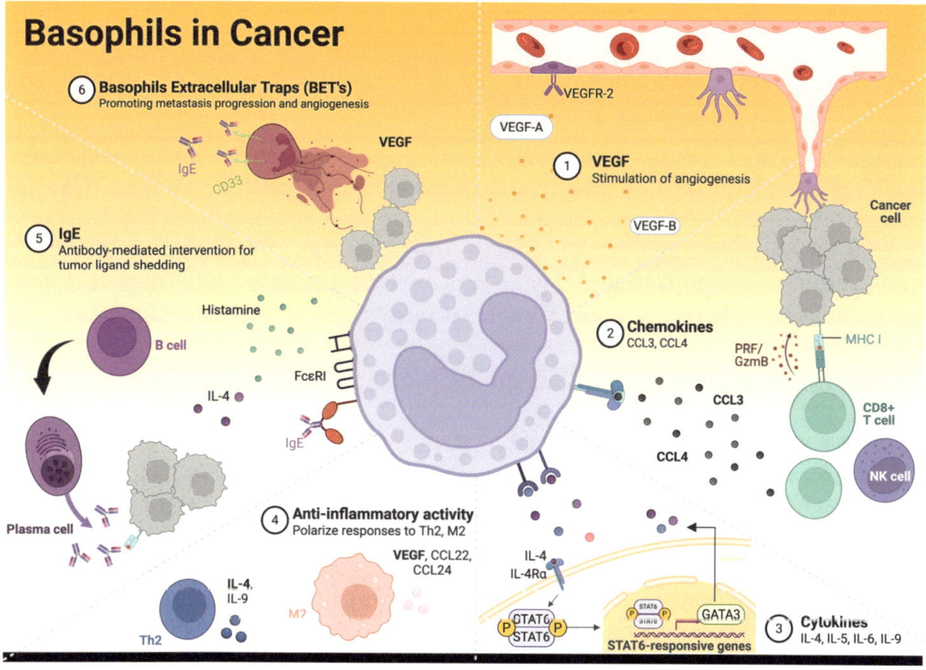

Figure 3.
Basophils in cancer. 1. VEGF. *Basophils release large amounts of VEGF-A and VEGF-B, which induce increased angiogenesis that can deliver nutrients to cancer cells and promote metastasis.* 2. Chemokines. *By releasing the chemokines CCL3 and CCL4, basophils induce the chemotaxis of cells such as CD8⁺ and NK cells, promoting immune infiltration and tumor regression. However, they can also attract M2 macrophages and Tregs, cells capable of promoting chronic inflammation and immunosuppression.* 3. Cytokines. *Cytokines such as IL-4 can trigger the JAK-STAT6 pathway, inducing immunosuppressive profiles in cells, promoting increased angiogenesis, and conferring resistance to apoptosis in certain tumors. It also stimulates B-cell and eosinophil-mediated responses, which, depending on the tumor, may contribute to increased metastasis or survival.* 4. Anti-inflammatory activity. *Basophils polarize lymphocyte and macrophage responses to Th2 and M2 profiles, which release large amounts of IL-4 and VEGF, creating an anti-inflammatory environment.* 5. Immunoglobulin E (IgE). *The binding of IgE to the FcεRI receptor can promote degranulation and the release of mediators such as histamine and IL-4. These stimulate the differentiation of B lymphocytes into plasma cells, which promotes greater IgE production. This interaction can have both anti- and pro-tumor effects.* 6. Basophils extracellular traps (BETs). *IgE secretion can induce the release of BETs, which can exert an antitumor effect by trapping cancer cells in their networks. However, their persistent formation could induce tissue damage and alterations in the extracellular matrix, favoring tumor invasion and dissemination. Created in https://BioRender.com.*

molecules such as IL-3 and VEGF, which stimulate the secretion of CCL3 and CCL4, favoring the infiltration of cytotoxic T cells. In contrast, in microenvironments dominated by Th2-type signals, galectin-3, interleukins IL-4 and IL-13 may contribute to immunosuppression and tumor growth.

From a clinical perspective, the presence of a higher concentration of activated basophils is associated with a better prognosis in cancers such as ovarian cancer, melanoma, and colorectal cancer [66, 72]. In contrast, in cancers such as pancreatic, chronic myeloid leukemia, lung, and gastric cancer, there is a higher risk of metastasis and lower survival [74–76]. Understanding how microenvironmental signals modulate basophil activity may offer novel strategies in cancer immunotherapy, maximizing their antitumor potential while minimizing protumor effects.

4.2 Basophils in breast cancer

In BC, growing evidence suggests that basophil presence and activation can significantly influence both tumor dynamics and clinical outcomes. A transcriptomic analysis of breast tumor samples revealed that higher expression of canonical basophil markers, such as CD123, CCR3, and FcεRI, was significantly associated with improved relapse-free survival (RFS) and overall survival (OS) in patients with BC. When stratified by tumor subtype, patients with ER-/HER-2- breast cancer showed more favorable OS over a 60-month follow-up period when exhibiting elevated basophil gene expression signatures [75]. These findings are particularly relevant for TNBC, a subtype with poor prognosis and limited treatment options.

Conversely, preclinical studies in mouse models have suggested a more important and potentially dual role for basophils in BC. In one murine model, the presence of basophils was associated with tumor growth. However, paradoxically, in cases where the basophil percentage (BASO%) was higher, particularly in mice with confirmed metastasis, the number of metastatic foci in the lungs was reduced [77]. This duality may reflect stage-specific or context-dependent basophil functions influenced by the tumor microenvironment and immune signaling landscape. Functionally, activated basophils are capable of releasing a wide range of cytotoxic and inflammatory mediators, including granzyme B, TNF-α, and histamine, which can act directly on tumor cells. Notably, histamine has been shown to improve survival in a mouse model of BC, suggesting a potential protective effect [72].

Moreover, basophils interact with other immune cells to enhance antitumor immunity. They have been reported to stimulate B cells through CD40L expression and the release of IL-4, IL-6, IL-13, BAFF, and histamine, all of which contribute to B cell proliferation, survival, and antibody-mediated responses against tumor cells. Together, these findings support the notion that basophils are not passive or only proinflammatory cells, but rather active participants in the immunobiology of breast cancer. **Figure 4** reflects his complexity, contrasting the worse prognosis associated with higher basophil concentrations in animal models against the improved survival linked to elevated basophil marker expression in clinical studies. Depending on the immune context and tumor subtype, their effects may be either tumor-promoting or tumor-suppressive, and their cytokine profile positions them as the promising prognostic biomarkers and potential targets for immunotherapeutic strategies.

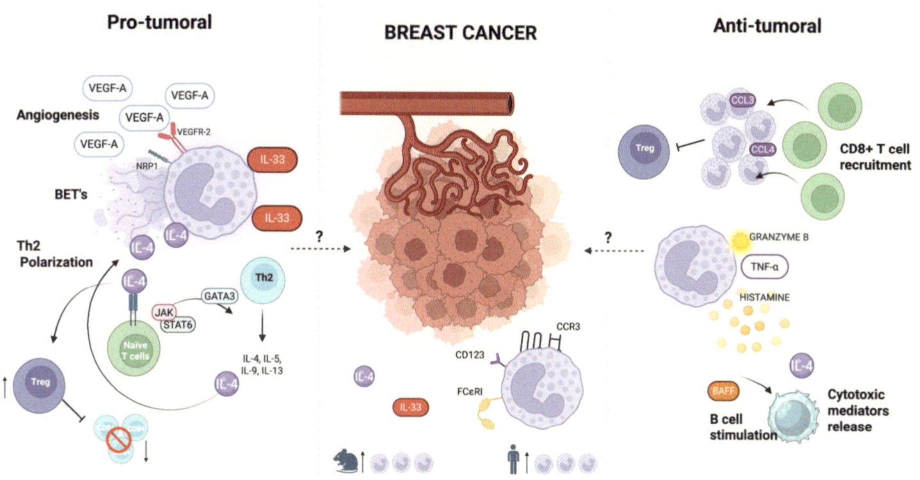

Figure 4.
Basophils and their activity in breast cancer. Although research has identified mechanisms by which basophils exert pro-tumorigenic and anti-tumorigenic effects, studies specifically investigating breast cancer remain limited. In animal models, elevated basophil concentrations are associated with a poorer prognosis. Conversely, clinical studies have found that increased expression of basophil-specific markers correlates with improved survival outcomes. Created in https://BioRender.com.

5. Treatment

5.1 Eosinophils as treatment for breast cancer

Eosinophils, traditionally recognized for their roles in allergic responses and parasitic infections, have recently garnered attention as key players in tumor immunology. Their influence on BC appears to be context-dependent, with the potential to either support or hinder tumor progression depending on the TME. This discussion highlights two key perspectives: eosinophils as effectors of antitumor immunity and as modulators within broader immunotherapeutic strategies (**Figure 5**). The insights are supported by evidence from both experimental models and human studies, offering a comprehensive understanding of their clinical potential.

5.1.1 Preclinical studies

In preclinical models, recent studies in mice have shown that estrogens can suppress eosinophilic responses in mammary tumors. Specifically, estradiol was found to reduce both systemic eosinophil levels and their infiltration into tumors. Using ovariectomized mice implanted with estrogen-dependent BC cells (A7C11, E0771), results demonstrated that blocking estrogen receptors with agents such as fulvestrant reinstated eosinophil presence in the tumor and led to significant tumor regression. Importantly, when eosinophils were experimentally depleted, the therapeutic benefit of anti-estrogen treatment was lost, suggesting that eosinophils are essential mediators in this response [78].

Complementary findings suggest that immune checkpoint inhibitors (ICIs), such as anti-PD1 and anti-CTLA-4, enhance IL-5-producing $CD4^+$ T cells, thereby promoting eosinophil generation in the bone marrow and subsequent migration to tumors.

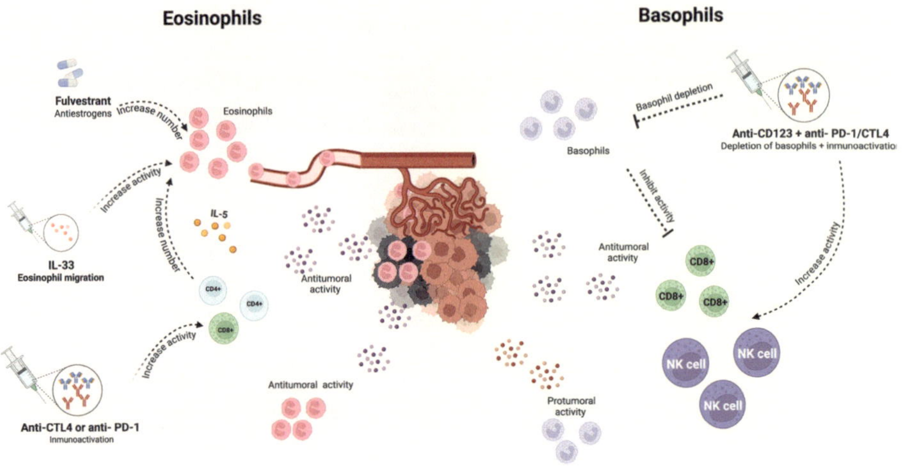

Figure 5.
Immunomodulatory roles of eosinophils and basophils in breast cancer treatment. Eosinophils: preclinical studies show that estrogen signaling suppresses eosinophilic activity in breast tumors, while treatments with anti-estrogen receptors restore their infiltration and contribute to tumor regression. Immune checkpoint inhibitors (anti-PD-1 and anti-CTLA-4) and IL-33 enhance eosinophil recruitment and interactions with $CD8^+$ and $CD4^+$ T cells, thereby further boosting antitumor effects. Clinically, treatment-induced eosinophilia has been associated with improved progression-free survival in breast cancer patients, suggesting that eosinophils may serve as both biomarkers and effectors of therapeutic success. Basophils are being investigated for their role in modulating the tumor immune microenvironment. Depletion strategies targeting basophils, such as anti-CD123 antibodies, enhance the efficacy of PD-1 or CTL4-treatment, increasing cytotoxic antitumor responses. Created in https://BioRender.com.

Administration of IL-33 further increased eosinophil infiltration and improved interactions with $CD8^+$ T cells, amplifying antitumor effects. Eosinophil depletion nullified these responses, reinforcing their crucial role in the ICIs efficacy [32]. Additional mechanistic studies have elucidated how eosinophil-derived cytokines, such as IL-5, GM-CSF, and IL-33, reconfigure the tumor microenvironment, facilitate T cell recruitment, and impede angiogenesis. Preliminary hypotheses also suggest potential synergy between eosinophils and CAR-T cell therapy, although this concept remains to be studied experimentally [79].

5.1.2 Clinical studies

In human studies, although eosinophils have not yet been directly targeted in clinical trials for BC, observational data suggest their involvement. In patients with metastatic TNBC receiving chemo-immunotherapy, those who developed eosinophilia during treatment exhibited better progression-free survival, implying a connection between eosinophil activity and immunotherapeutic success. Further analysis of tumor and blood samples from patients treated with ICIs revealed increased eosinophil levels both peripherally and within tumors, particularly in those who experienced clinical benefit. These findings were accompanied by elevated expression of IL-5 and IL-33, mirroring trends observed in murine studies and highlighting eosinophil activation as a marker and mediator of therapeutic response [32].

Currently, no clinical trials are investigating the use of eosinophil-targeted cytokines, such as IL-5 or IL-33 agonists, in BC. However, drugs that modulate eosinophil activity, such as anti-IL-5 monoclonal antibodies (mepolizumab, benralizumab), have been safely administered in other diseases. These treatments demonstrate that eosinophils are clinically accessible and modifiable targets, highlighting their potential for future cancer-focused applications.

5.2 Basophils as treatment for breast and other cancers

The ability of basophils to secrete cytokines such as IL-4 and histamine, and their expression of receptors including FcεRI, CD123, and CCR3, make them an important target for the development of targeted therapies in cancer treatment. **Figure 5** summarizes that both eosinophils and basophils can be modulated through approaches such as checkpoint inhibitors, anti-estrogen treatments, or anti-CD123 strategies to shift the immune balance toward antitumor activity in breast cancer. A recent study investigated the clinical efficacy of IgE immunotherapy utilizing the monoclonal antibody IgE MOv18, which targets the folate receptor α, a protein overexpressed in certain epithelial tumors. The findings of this study indicate a positive correlation between antibody administration and the presence of antitumor activity [80]. Given the expression of the FcεRI receptor, basophils could be therapeutically modulated in oncology, contributing to an effective antitumor immune response, particularly in cancers such as ovarian or even breast cancer with high expression of CD123, CCR3, and FcεRI.

Another strategy that could be addressed is the blockade of pro-tumor mediators secreted by basophils, such as IL-4 and histamine. A study conducted in mice with lung cancer found that the specific deletion of the IL-4Rα protein in early myeloid progenitors in the bone marrow was capable of inducing a decrease in tumor burden [74]. Clinically, the administration of dupilumab, an IL-4Rα blocker, and anti-PD-L1 yielded results consistent with the murine models: a reduction in circulating monocytes and an increase in $CD8^+$ T cells infiltrating the tumor. Similar results were identified with anti-IL-4 antibodies [81]. Furthermore, histamine H1 receptor antagonists, such as azelastine and terfenadine, have been shown to reduce the activation of cancer-associated fibroblasts, decrease STAT3 signaling, and enhance the response to anti-PD-1 treatments [82, 83].

A recent proposal is the direct depletion of the basophil population using anti-CD123, which could reduce chronic inflammation, restore $CD8^+$ T cell and NK cell activity, and improve the efficacy of therapies such as anti-PD-1/PD-L1 [84]. However, it could also decrease the antitumor immune response, so therapies aimed at basophil depletion must be specific enough to distinguish between an immunosuppressive environment and one that cooperates with the antitumor response. Moreover, the technical difficulty of isolating and expanding human basophils *in vitro* under clinical conditions. To identify these discrepancies in immuno-oncology, researchers can utilize the Basophil Activation Test (BAT), a test that evaluates the activation of basophils in peripheral blood in response to specific stimuli to monitor the safety of novel, personalized therapies and study the function of basophils in oncology patients [85].

In the future, clinical efforts could focus on developing dual strategies: on the one hand, inhibiting the function of basophils when they promote immunosuppression or chronic tumor inflammation, and on the other hand, enhancing their effector capacity in contexts where they exert immunostimulatory functions. Simultaneously, the use of tests such as the BAT could optimize the selection and monitoring of patients in personalized immunological therapies.

6. Conclusions

Eosinophils and basophils are underestimated leukocytes. Although their presence within the tumor was described more than 100 years ago, their role in cancer and the mechanisms involved in the pro- or antitumoral activities have been recently elucidated. Although the number of these cells is low, circulating or within the tumor, the presence of eosinophils serves as a favorable prognostic factor in contexts such as bladder, colorectal, and prostate cancers. Conversely, it correlates with tumor progression in melanoma and non-small-cell lung cancer. Similarly, activated basophils are linked to improved prognoses in ovarian, melanoma, and colorectal cancers. In contrast, in pancreatic, chronic myeloid leukemia, lung, and gastric cancers, they indicate a higher risk of metastasis and decreased survival.

Functionally, both cell types possess a large number of cytotoxic molecules that can act directly to destroy cancer cells. Still, they can also act indirectly by releasing cytokines and other soluble factors that modulate the TME. Moreover, this modulation can have a synergistic effect in some new immune checkpoint blockade therapies, where eosinophils can promote the efficient activation of $CD8^+$ cells, and the concomitant administration of chemotherapy and alarmins, such as IL-33, can improve overall response and survival. For basophils, the landscape is unclear, and depletion of these cells is suggested.

The ongoing clinical efforts could focus on developing dual strategies: enhancing the antitumoral capacity of eosinophils and basophils and promoting the infiltration of these cells within the tumor to optimize the selection of effective immune cells and create a microenvironment that blocks the progression of BC. The role of these cells as a TME component in the regulation of antitumor immunity and ICI response has been elucidated. Whether an increase in eosinophils or basophils could be used as a biomarker of treatment efficacy and/or lead to the development of new therapeutic avenues in breast and other tumors needs to be further studied to offer personalized and more effective immunological therapies.

The goal of this chapter is to provide an overview of the role of these cells in cancer, with a specific focus on breast cancer, and their involvement in disease progression. These cells and their associated markers may represent potential therapeutic targets, particularly in cases where conventional treatments are ineffective. Furthermore, the scarcity of information on these cells in the context of cancer highlights the need for further research, as they may serve as indicators of treatment efficacy.

Conflict of interest

The authors declare no conflict of interest.

Author details

Claudia A. Garay-Canales[1], Raul Aragon-Franco[1], Yair Rodríguez-Santiago[1], Diana L. Ruiz-Antonio[1,2], María del Sol Ríos-Avila[3,4], César A. Zavala-López[3,4], Karen E. Nava-Castro[3] and Jorge Morales-Montor[1]*

1 Immunology Department, Instituto de Investigaciones Biomédicas, Universidad Nacional Autónoma de México, Mexico City, Mexico

2 Posgrado en Ciencias Bioquímicas, Universidad Nacional Autónoma de México, Mexico City, Mexico

3 Department of Atmospheric Science, Instituto de Ciencias de la Atmósfera y Cambio Climático, Universidad Nacional Autónoma de México, Mexico City, Mexico

4 Posgrado en Ciencias Biológicas, Universidad Nacional Autónoma de México, Mexico City, Mexico

*Address all correspondence to: jmontor66@iibiomedicas.unam.mx

References

[1] Terry MB, Colditz GA. Epidemiology and risk factors for breast cancer: 21st century advances, gaps to address through interdisciplinary science. Cold Spring Harbor Perspectives in Medicine. 2023;**13**:a041317. DOI: 10.1101/cshperspect.a041317

[2] GLOBOCAN. Global Cancer Burden in 2022. Global Cancer Today. Lyon: GLOBOCAN; 2022. Available from: https://gco.iarc.fr/today/en/dataviz/tables [Accessed: May 27, 2025]

[3] Esquivel-Velázquez M, Ostoa-Saloma P, Palacios-Arreola MI, Nava-Castro KE, Castro JI, Morales-Montor J. The role of cytokines in breast cancer development and progression. Journal of Interferon & Cytokine Research: The Official Journal of the International Society for Interferon and Cytokine Research. 2015;**35**:1-16. DOI: 10.1089/jir.2014.0026

[4] Bhardwaj PV, Gupta S, Elyash A, Teplinsky E. Male breast cancer: A review on diagnosis, treatment, and survivorship. Current Oncology Reports. 2024;**26**:34-45. DOI: 10.1007/s11912-023-01489-z

[5] Chidambaram A, Prabhakaran R, Sivasamy S, Kanagasabai T, Thekkumalai M, Singh A, et al. Male breast cancer: Current scenario and future perspectives. Technology in Cancer Research & Treatment. 2024;**23**:15330338241261836. DOI: 10.1177/15330338241261836

[6] Herrera-Quintana L, Vázquez-Lorente H, Plaza-Diaz J. Breast cancer: Extracellular matrix and microbiome interactions. International Journal of Molecular Sciences. 2024;**25**:7226. DOI: 10.3390/ijms25137226

[7] Carvalho E, Canberk S, Schmitt F, Vale N. Molecular subtypes and mechanisms of breast cancer: Precision medicine approaches for targeted therapies. Cancers. 2025;**17**:1102. DOI: 10.3390/cancers17071102

[8] Xiong X, Zheng L-W, Ding Y, Chen Y-F, Cai Y-W, Wang L-P, et al. Breast cancer: Pathogenesis and treatments. Signal Transduction and Targeted Therapy. 2025;**10**:49. DOI: 10.1038/s41392-024-02108-4

[9] Barzaman K, Karami J, Zarei Z, Hosseinzadeh A, Kazemi MH, Moradi-Kalbolandi S, et al. Breast cancer: Biology, biomarkers, and treatments. International Immunopharmacology. 2020;**84**:106535. DOI: 10.1016/j.intimp.2020.106535

[10] Artham S, Chang C-Y, McDonnell DP. Eosinophilia in cancer and its regulation by sex hormones. Trends in Endocrinology and Metabolism: TEM. 2023;**34**:5-20. DOI: 10.1016/j.tem.2022.11.002

[11] Gigon L, Fettrelet T, Yousefi S, Simon D, Simon H. Eosinophils from A to Z. Allergy. 2023;**78**:1810-1846. DOI: 10.1111/all.15751

[12] Lacy P, Rosenberg HF, Walsh GM. Molecular biology of eosinophils: Introduction. In: Eosinophils. New York, NY: Humana; 2021. pp. 1-14. DOI: 10.1007/978-1-0716-1095-4_1

[13] Omman RA, Kini AR. Leukocyte development, kinetics, and functions. In: Rodak's Hematology. Missouri: Elsevier; 2020. pp. 117-135. DOI: 10.1016/B978-0-323-53045-3.00018-0

[14] Poto R, Loffredo S, Marone G, Di Salvatore A, de Paulis A, Schroeder JT, et al. Basophils beyond allergic

and parasitic diseases. Frontiers in Immunology. 2023;**14**:1190034. DOI: 10.3389/fimmu.2023.1190034

[15] Siracusa MC. Basophils – Role in immunity. In: Encyclopedia of Immunobiology. Oxford: Elsevier; 2016. pp. 326-333. DOI: 10.1016/B978-0-12-374279-7.03006-X

[16] Varricchi G, Raap U, Rivellese F, Marone G, Gibbs BF. Human mast cells and basophils—How are they similar how are they different? Immunological Reviews. 2018;**282**:8-34. DOI: 10.1111/imr.12627

[17] Place AE, Jin Huh S, Polyak K. The microenvironment in breast cancer progression: Biology and implications for treatment. Breast Cancer Research: BCR. 2011;**13**:227. DOI: 10.1186/bcr2912

[18] Rodríguez-Bejarano OH, Parra-López C, Patarroyo MA. A review concerning the breast cancer-related tumour microenvironment. Critical Reviews in Oncology/Hematology. 2024;**199**:104389. DOI: 10.1016/j.critrevonc.2024.104389

[19] Li JJ, Tsang JY, Tse GM. Tumor microenvironment in breast cancer—Updates on therapeutic implications and pathologic assessment. Cancers. 2021;**13**:4233. DOI: 10.3390/cancers13164233

[20] Harris MA, Savas P, Virassamy B, O'Malley MMR, Kay J, Mueller SN, et al. Towards targeting the breast cancer immune microenvironment. Nature Reviews. Cancer. 2024;**24**:554-577. DOI: 10.1038/s41568-024-00714-6

[21] Otterlei Fjørtoft M, Huse K, Rye IH. The tumor immune microenvironment in breast cancer progression. Acta Oncologica. 2024;**63**:33008. DOI: 10.2340/1651-226X.2024.33008

[22] Garay-Canales CA, Segovia-Mendoza M, Rodríguez-Santiago Y, Nava-Castro KE, Ríos-Avila MDS, López GEÁ, et al. Advances in intratumoral immunotherapy from a neuro-immune-endocrine perspective for breast cancer treatment. Frontiers in Oncology. 2026;**16**:1735300. DOI: 10.3389/fonc.2026.1735300

[23] Roma-Rodrigues C, Mendes R, Baptista PV, Fernandes AR. Targeting tumor microenvironment for cancer therapy. International Journal of Molecular Sciences. 2019;**20**:840. DOI: 10.3390/ijms20040840

[24] Ruffell B, Au A, Rugo HS, Esserman LJ, Hwang ES, Coussens LM. Leukocyte composition of human breast cancer. Proceedings of the National Academy of Sciences. 2012;**109**:2796-2801. DOI: 10.1073/pnas.1104303108

[25] DeNardo DG, Coussens LM. Inflammation and breast cancer. Balancing immune response: Crosstalk between adaptive and innate immune cells during breast cancer progression. Breast Cancer Research. 2007;**9**:212. DOI: 10.1186/bcr1746

[26] Dushyanthen S, Beavis PA, Savas P, Teo ZL, Zhou C, Mansour M, et al. Relevance of tumor-infiltrating lymphocytes in breast cancer. BMC Medicine. 2015;**13**:202. DOI: 10.1186/s12916-015-0431-3

[27] Stanton SE, Disis ML. Clinical significance of tumor-infiltrating lymphocytes in breast cancer. Journal for Immunotherapy of Cancer. 2016;**4**:59. DOI: 10.1186/s40425-016-0165-6

[28] Fukui R, Fujimoto Y, Watanabe T, Inoue N, Bun A, Higuchi T, et al. Association between FOXP3/CD8 lymphocyte ratios and tumor infiltrating lymphocyte levels in different breast

cancer subtypes. Anticancer Research. 2020;**40**:2141-2150. DOI: 10.21873/anticanres.14173

[29] Stanton SE, Adams S, Disis ML. Variation in the incidence and magnitude of tumor-infiltrating lymphocytes in breast cancer subtypes: A systematic review. JAMA Oncology. 2016;**2**:1354-1360. DOI: 10.1001/jamaoncol.2016.1061

[30] Kim HM, Koo JS. Clinicopathologic characteristics of breast cancer according to the infiltrating immune cell subtypes. International Journal of Molecular Sciences. 2020;**21**:4438. DOI: 10.3390/ijms21124438

[31] Sadeghalvad M, Mohammadi-Motlagh H-R, Rezaei N. Immune microenvironment in different molecular subtypes of ductal breast carcinoma. Breast Cancer Research and Treatment. 2021;**185**:261-279. DOI: 10.1007/s10549-020-05954-2

[32] Blomberg OS, Spagnuolo L, Garner H, Voorwerk L, Isaeva OI, van Dyk E, et al. IL-5-producing CD4+ T cells and eosinophils cooperate to enhance response to immune checkpoint blockade in breast cancer. Cancer Cell. 2023;**41**:106-123.e10. DOI: 10.1016/j.ccell.2022.11.014

[33] Kay AB. The early history of the eosinophil. Clinical and Experimental Allergy. 2015;**45**:575-582. DOI: 10.1111/cea.12480

[34] Kay AB. Paul Ehrlich and the early history of granulocytes. Microbiology Spectrum. 2016;**4**:4. DOI: 10.1128/microbiolspec.mchd-0032-2016

[35] Valent P, Groner B, Schumacher U, Superti-Furga G, Busslinger M, Kralovics R, et al. Paul Ehrlich (1854-1915) and his contributions to the foundation and birth of translational medicine. Journal of Innate Immunity. 2016;**8**:111-120. DOI: 10.1159/000443526

[36] Tamaki M, Konno Y, Kobayashi Y, Takeda M, Itoga M, Moritoki Y, et al. Expression and functional roles of G-protein-coupled estrogen receptor (GPER) in human eosinophils. Immunology Letters. 2014;**160**:72-78. DOI: 10.1016/j.imlet.2014.03.012

[37] Hogan SP, Rosenberg HF, Moqbel R, Phipps S, Foster PS, Lacy P, et al. Eosinophils: Biological properties and role in health and disease. Clinical and Experimental Allergy. 2008;**38**:709-750. DOI: 10.1111/j.1365-2222.2008.02958.x

[38] Araújo JMD, Silva LAS, Felix FB, Camargo EA, Grespan R. CCR3 antagonist impairs estradiol-induced eosinophil migration to the uterus in ovariectomized mice. Brazilian Journal of Medical and Biological Research. 2019;**53**:e8659. DOI: 10.1590/1414-431X20198659

[39] Hamano N, Terada N, Maesako K-I, Numata T, Konno A. Effect of sex hormones on eosinophilic inflammation in nasal mucosa. Allergy and Asthma Proceedings. 1998;**19**:263-269. DOI: 10.2500/108854198778557773

[40] vom Steeg LG, Dhakal S, Woldetsadik YA, Park H-S, Mulka KR, Reilly EC, et al. Androgen receptor signaling in the lungs mitigates inflammation and improves the outcome of influenza in mice. PLoS Pathogens. 2020;**16**:e1008506. DOI: 10.1371/journal.ppat.1008506

[41] Gouon-Evans V, Lin EY, Pollard JW. Requirement of macrophages and eosinophils and their cytokines/chemokines for mammary gland development. Breast Cancer Research. 2002;**4**:155. DOI: 10.1186/bcr441

[42] Gatault S, Legrand F, Delbeke M, Loiseau S, Capron M. Involvement of eosinophils in the anti-tumor response. Cancer Immunology, Immunotherapy. 2012;**61**:1527-1534. DOI: 10.1007/s00262-012-1288-3

[43] Day KS, Rempel L, Rossi FMV, Theret M. Origins and functions of eosinophils in two non-mucosal tissues. Frontiers in Immunology. 2024;**15**:1368142. DOI: 10.3389/fimmu.2024.1368142

[44] Reichman H, Karo-Atar D, Munitz A. Emerging roles for eosinophils in the tumor microenvironment. Trends Cancer. 2016;**2**:664-675. DOI: 10.1016/j.trecan.2016.10.002

[45] Simon SCS, Utikal J, Umansky V. Opposing roles of eosinophils in cancer. Cancer Immunology, Immunotherapy. 2019;**68**:823-833. DOI: 10.1007/s00262-018-2255-4

[46] Leighton SEJ, Teo JGC, Leung SF, Cheung AYK, Lee JCK, Van Hasselt CA. Prevalence and prognostic significance of tumor-associated tissue eosinophilia in nasopharyngeal carcinoma. Cancer. 1996;**77**:436-440. DOI: 10.1002/(sici)1097-0142(19960201)77:3%253C436::aid-cncr3%253E3.0.co;2-i

[47] Samoszuk MK, Nguyen V, Gluzman I, Pham JH. Occult deposition of eosinophil peroxidase in a subset of human breast carcinomas. The American Journal of Pathology. 1996;**148**:701-706

[48] Szalayova G, Ogrodnik A, Spencer B, Wade J, Bunn J, Ambaye A, et al. Human breast cancer biopsies induce eosinophil recruitment and enhance adjacent cancer cell proliferation. Breast Cancer Research and Treatment. 2016;**157**:461-474. DOI: 10.1007/s10549-016-3839-3

[49] Grisaru-Tal S, Itan M, Grass DG, Torres-Roca J, Eschrich SA, Gordon Y, et al. Primary tumors from mucosal barrier organs drive unique eosinophil infiltration patterns and clinical associations. Oncoimmunology. 2021;**10**:e1859732. DOI: 10.1080/2162402x.2020.1859732

[50] Ali HR, Chlon L, Pharoah PDP, Markowetz F, Caldas C. Patterns of immune infiltration in breast cancer and their clinical implications: A gene-expression-based retrospective study. PLoS Medicine. 2016;**13**:e1002194. DOI: 10.1371/journal.pmed.1002194

[51] Chouliaras K, Tokumaru Y, Asaoka M, Oshi M, Attwood KM, Yoshida K, et al. Prevalence and clinical relevance of tumor-associated tissue eosinophilia (TATE) in breast cancer. Surgery. 2021;**169**:1234-1239. DOI: 10.1016/j.surg.2020.07.052

[52] Hollande C, Boussier J, Ziai J, Nozawa T, Bondet V, Phung W, et al. Inhibition of the dipeptidyl peptidase DPP4 (CD26) reveals IL-33-dependent eosinophil-mediated control of tumor growth. Nature Immunology. 2019;**20**:257-264. DOI: 10.1038/s41590-019-0321-5

[53] Sokol CL, Medzhitov R. Emerging functions of basophils in protective and allergic immune responses. Mucosal Immunology. 2010;**3**:129-137. DOI: 10.1038/mi.2009.137

[54] Nakashima C, Otsuka A, Kabashima K. Recent advancement in the mechanism of basophil activation. Journal of Dermatological Science. 2018;**91**:3-8. DOI: 10.1016/j.jdermsci.2018.03.007

[55] Shah H, Eisenbarth S, Tormey CA, Siddon AJ. Behind the scenes with basophils: An emerging therapeutic target. Immunotherapy Advances. 2021;**1**:ltab008. DOI: 10.1093/immadv/ltab008

[56] Cocchiara R, Albeggiani G, Di Trapani G, Azzolina A, Lampiasi N, Rizzo F, et al. Modulation of rat peritoneal mast cell and human basophil histamine release by estrogens. International Archives of Allergy and Immunology. 1990;**93**:192-197. DOI: 10.1159/000235300

[57] Zaitsu M, Narita S-I, Lambert KC, Grady JJ, Estes DM, Curran EM, et al. Estradiol activates mast cells via a non-genomic estrogen receptor-α and calcium influx. Molecular Immunology. 2007;**44**:1977-1985. DOI: 10.1016/j.molimm.2006.09.030

[58] De Paulis A, Prevete N, Fiorentino I, Rossi FW, Staibano S, Montuori N, et al. Expression and functions of the vascular endothelial growth factors and their receptors in human basophils. Journal of Immunology. 2006;**177**:7322-7331. DOI: 10.4049/jimmunol.177.10.7322

[59] Cao Y. Antiangiogenic cancer therapy. Seminars in Cancer Biology. 2004;**14**:139-145. DOI: 10.1016/j.semcancer.2003.09.018

[60] Yang Y, Cao Y. The impact of VEGF on cancer metastasis and systemic disease. Seminars in Cancer Biology. 2022;**86**:251-261. DOI: 10.1016/j.semcancer.2022.03.011

[61] Mabeta P, Steenkamp V. The VEGF/VEGFR axis revisited: Implications for cancer therapy. International Journal of Molecular Sciences. 2022;**23**:15585. DOI: 10.3390/ijms232415585

[62] Sharma S, Ehrlich M, Zhang M, Blobe GC, Henis YI. NRP1 interacts with endoglin and VEGFR2 to modulate VEGF signaling and endothelial cell sprouting. Communications Biology. 2024;**7**:112. DOI: 10.1038/s42003-024-05798-2

[63] Yoshimoto T, Yasuda K, Tanaka H, Nakahira M, Imai Y, Fujimori Y, et al. Basophils contribute to TH2-IgE responses in vivo via IL-4 production and presentation of peptide–MHC class II complexes to CD4+ T cells. Nature Immunology. 2009;**10**:706-712. DOI: 10.1038/ni.1737

[64] Poddighe D, Mathias CB, Freyschmidt EJ, Kombe D, Caplan B, Marseglia GL, et al. Basophils are rapidly mobilized following initial aeroallergen encounter in naïve mice and provide a priming source of IL-4 in adaptive immune responses. Journal of Biological Regulators and Homeostatic Agents. 2014;**28**:91-103

[65] Yamanishi Y, Miyake K, Iki M, Tsutsui H, Karasuyama H. Recent advances in understanding basophil-mediated Th2 immune responses. Immunological Reviews. 2017;**278**:237-245. DOI: 10.1111/imr.12548

[66] Chauhan J, Stavraka C, Grandits M, Palhares LCGF, Josephs DH, Lacy KE, et al. Clinical and translational significance of basophils in patients with cancer. Cells. 2022;**11**:438. DOI: 10.3390/cells11030438

[67] Morshed M, Hlushchuk R, Simon D, Walls AF, Obata-Ninomiya K, Karasuyama H, et al. NADPH oxidase–independent formation of extracellular DNA traps by basophils. Journal of Immunology. 2014;**192**:5314-5323. DOI: 10.4049/jimmunol.1303418

[68] Park J, Wysocki RW, Amoozgar Z, Maiorino L, Fein MR, Jorns J, et al. Cancer cells induce metastasis-supporting neutrophil extracellular DNA traps. Science Translational Medicine. 2016;**8**:361ra138. DOI: 10.1126/scitranslmed.aag1711

[69] Albrengues J, Shields MA, Ng D, Park CG, Ambrico A, Poindexter ME, et al. Neutrophil extracellular traps produced during inflammation awaken dormant cancer cells in mice. Science. 2018;**361**:eaao4227. DOI: 10.1126/science.aao4227

[70] Poto R, Cristinziano L, Modestino L, De Paulis A, Marone G, Loffredo S, et al. Neutrophil extracellular traps, angiogenesis and cancer. Biomedicine. 2022;**10**:431. DOI: 10.3390/biomedicines10020431

[71] Sektioglu IM, Carretero R, Bulbuc N, Bald T, Tüting T, Rudensky AY, et al. Basophils promote tumor rejection via chemotaxis and infiltration of CD8+ T cells. Cancer Research. 2017;**77**:291-302. DOI: 10.1158/0008-5472.can-16-0993

[72] Bax HJ, Chauhan J, Stavraka C, Khiabany A, Nakamura M, Pellizzari G, et al. Basophils from cancer patients respond to immune stimuli and predict clinical outcome. Cells. 2020;**9**:1631. DOI: 10.3390/cells9071631

[73] Marone G, Gambardella AR, Mattei F, Mancini J, Schiavoni G, Varricchi G. Basophils in tumor microenvironment and surroundings. In: Advances in Experimental Medicine and Biology. Cham: Springer International Publishing; 2020. pp. 21-34. DOI: 10.1007/978-3-030-35723-8_2

[74] LaMarche NM, Hegde S, Park MD, Maier BB, Troncoso L, Le Berichel J, et al. An IL-4 signalling axis in bone marrow drives pro-tumorigenic myelopoiesis. Nature. 2024;**625**:166-174. DOI: 10.1038/s41586-023-06797-9

[75] He X, Cao Y, Gu Y, Fang H, Wang J, Liu X, et al. Clinical outcomes and immune metrics in intratumoral basophil-enriched gastric cancer patients. Annals of Surgical Oncology. 2021;**28**:6439-6450. DOI: 10.1245/s10434-021-09815-0

[76] Baba T, Tanabe Y, Yoshikawa S, Yamanishi Y, Morishita S, Komatsu N, et al. MIP-1α/CCL3-expressing basophil-lineage cells drive the leukemic hematopoiesis of chronic myeloid leukemia in mice. Blood. 2016;**127**:2607-2617. DOI: 10.1182/blood-2015-10-673087

[77] Wang C, Chen Y-G, Gao J-L, Lyu G-Y, Su J, Zhang Q, et al. Low local blood perfusion, high white blood cell and high platelet count are associated with primary tumor growth and lung metastasis in a 4T1 mouse breast cancer metastasis model. Oncology Letters. 2015;**10**:754-760. DOI: 10.3892/ol.2015.3304

[78] Artham S, Juras PK, Goyal A, Chakraborty P, Byemerwa J, Liu S, et al. Estrogen signaling suppresses tumor-associated tissue eosinophilia to promote breast tumor growth. Science Advances. 2024;**10**:eadp2442. DOI: 10.1126/sciadv.adp2442

[79] Ghaffari S, Rezaei N. Eosinophils in the tumor microenvironment: Implications for cancer immunotherapy. Journal of Translational Medicine. 2023;**21**:551. DOI: 10.1186/s12967-023-04418-7

[80] Spicer J, Basu B, Montes A, Banerji U, Kristeleit R, Miller R, et al. Safety and anti-tumour activity of the IgE antibody MOv18 in patients with advanced solid tumours expressing folate receptor-alpha: A phase I trial. Nature Communications. 2023;**14**:4180. DOI: 10.1038/s41467-023-39679-9

[81] Ito S, Shirota H, Kasahara Y, Saijo K, Ishioka C. IL-4 blockade alters the tumor microenvironment and augments the

response to cancer immunotherapy in a mouse model. Cancer Immunology, Immunotherapy. 2017;**66**:1485-1496. DOI: 10.1007/s00262-017-2043-6

[82] Baniya MK, Kim E-H, Chun K-S. Terfenadine, a histamine H1 receptor antagonist, induces apoptosis by suppressing STAT3 signaling in human colorectal cancer HCT116 cells. Frontiers in Pharmacology. 2024;**15**:1418266. DOI: 10.3389/fphar.2024.1418266

[83] Zhong P, Nakata K, Oyama K, Higashijima N, Sagara A, Date S, et al. Blockade of histamine receptor H1 augments immune checkpoint therapy by enhancing MHC-I expression in pancreatic cancer cells. Journal of Experimental & Clinical Cancer Research. 2024;**43**:138. DOI: 10.1186/s13046-024-03060-5

[84] Gauthier L, Virone-Oddos A, Beninga J, Rossi B, Nicolazzi C, Amara C, et al. Control of acute myeloid leukemia by a trifunctional NKp46-CD16a-NK cell engager targeting CD123. Nature Biotechnology. 2023;**41**:1296-1306. DOI: 10.1038/s41587-022-01626-2

[85] Sanz ML, Gamboa PM, Mayorga C. Basophil activation tests in the evaluation of immediate drug hypersensitivity. Current Opinion in Allergy and Clinical Immunology. 2009;**9**:298-304. DOI: 10.1097/aci.0b013e32832d5311